DATE DUE

OCT 2 6 1994	OCT 1 3 2000
NOV 1 0 1994	
NOV 2 3 1994	OCT 2 9 2002
1 2 1994	MAR 0 4 2003
FEB - 2 1995	
MAR - 2 1995	
MAR 1 6 1995	
MAR 2 8 1995	
APR 1 8 1995	
NOV 1 6 1995	
FEB 1 9 1996	
MAR 1 5 1996	
APR - 9 1996	
APR 2 1 1997	
NOV 2 3 1998	
DEC 1 1 1998	
OCT 1 7 1999	

BRODART

Cat. No. 23-221

Cocaine

Second Edition

Cocaine

Second Edition

Roger D. Weiss, M.D.
Steven M. Mirin, M.D.
Roxanne L. Bartel, M.D.

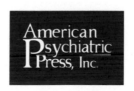

Washington, DC
London, England

Note: The authors have worked to ensure that all information in this book concerning drug dosages, schedules, and routes of administration is accurate as of the time of publication and consistent with standards set by the U.S. Food and Drug Administration and the general medical community. As medical research and practice advance, however, therapeutic standards may change. For this reason and because human and mechanical errors sometimes occur, we recommend that readers follow the advice of a physician who is directly involved in their care or the care of a member of their family.

Books published by the American Psychiatric Press, Inc., represent the views and opinions of the individual authors and do not necessarily represent the policies and opinions of the Press or the American Psychiatric Association.

Copyright © 1994 Roger D. Weiss, Steven M. Mirin,
and Roxanne L. Bartel
ALL RIGHTS RESERVED
Manufactured in the United States of America on acid-free paper
97 96 95 94   4 3 2 1
Second Edition

American Psychiatric Press, Inc.
1400 K Street, N.W., Washington, DC   20005

Library of Congress Cataloging-in-Publication Data
Weiss, Roger D., 1951–
    Cocaine / Roger D. Weiss, Steven M. Mirin, and Roxanne L. Bartel.
        p.   cm.
    Includes bibliographical references and index.
    ISBN 0-88048-549-3
    1. Cocaine habit. 2. Cocaine—Physiological effect. I. Mirin,
StevenM., 1942–   . II. Bartel, Roxanne L.   III. Title.
    [DNLM: 1. Cocaine. 2. Substance Abuse. WM280 W432c 1994]
    RC568.C6W46   1994
    616.8647—dc20
    DNLM/DLC
    for Library of Congress   93-15802
                                                                              CIP

British Library Cataloguing in Publication Data
A CIP record is available from the British Library.

To our families,
with love and appreciation

Contents

About the Authors

Roger D. Weiss, M.D., is Clinical Director of the Alcohol and Drug Abuse Program at McLean Hospital in Belmont, Massachusetts, and Associate Professor of Psychiatry at Harvard Medical School. Steven M. Mirin, M.D., is General Director and Psychiatrist in Chief at McLean Hospital and Professor of Psychiatry at Harvard Medical School. Roxanne L. Bartel, M.D., is Clinical Instructor in Psychiatry at the University of Utah in Salt Lake City, Utah.

Preface

Cocaine use remains one of the major public health and social problems in the United States today. The 1991 Household Survey conducted by the National Institute on Drug Abuse reported that 23 million Americans had used cocaine at some point during their lives. Medical complications and deaths from cocaine have continued to rise dramatically during the past decade. The popularity of cocaine has spawned and supported a huge illegal network dedicated to its manufacture, importation, and distribution. The cost of cocaine use to industry in lost productivity, job-related accidents, claims for health care benefits, and poor employee morale is likely billions of dollars a year. The personal cost to cocaine users, their families, and their friends is incalculable.

Much has been learned since we wrote the First Edition of *Cocaine*. Scientists have clarified how the drug works, and we have come to understand much more clearly both the short-term and long-term effects of cocaine on the brain and on the rest of the body. Patterns of cocaine use have changed, since the introduction of "crack" has increased the popularity of smoking cocaine. Treatment has changed as well, as a tremendous research effort has been mounted to discover the most effective ways to help cocaine-dependent patients. In this Second Edition of *Cocaine,* we have highlighted these recent developments in the use of cocaine and its treatment.

Our mission in writing the Second Edition of *Cocaine* remains the same: to provide a comprehensive overview of the subject of cocaine use. This book is written for those whose lives have been, or may be, affected by cocaine and for those who treat cocaine users. In this book we discuss what cocaine is, the different methods of its use, its effects on the brain and other organs, and its psychological and social consequences for users and those around them, both at home and in the workplace. We also discuss cocaine dependence (addiction)—how it happens, who is at risk, how to treat it, and how to find help. *Cocaine* includes a list of commonly asked questions about cocaine and a self-test for cocaine dependence.

Much of what we have learned about cocaine use has been gained through our experience working with patients on the Alcohol and Drug Abuse Treatment Center at McLean Hospital in Belmont, Massachusetts. We are grateful to the staff who have worked so hard to make that program successful and to the patients who have shared their experiences with us. In relating those experiences here, we have changed the names of our patients and other details about their lives to protect their anonymity.

Finally, we are grateful to Scott Lukas and Arthur Siegel, who reviewed sections of the book and contributed helpful comments; Cathryn Hufford, who helped track down the most current data available on cocaine; and Marjorie Maxwell, who worked tirelessly and enthusiastically on the manuscript through its many revisions. One of us (RDW) has received support from National Institute on Drug Abuse Grants DA05944 and U18 DA07693, which have been critical in allowing us to complete this second edition. We are also grateful to The Charles Engelhard Foundation for its long-standing support of the clinical research component of our program.

Roger D. Weiss, M.D.
Steven M. Mirin, M.D.
Roxanne L. Bartel, M.D.

Chapter 1

The Current Cocaine Epidemic

The Scope of the Problem

As we approach the 21st century, cocaine abuse remains a major public health problem in the United States. Most people today are aware of the dangers of cocaine addiction, and as a result occasional use of cocaine has decreased. On the other hand, more individuals are using cocaine frequently and in greater amounts, which has led to an increase in medical complications and deaths due to cocaine overdose, drug-related crime, and cocaine use during pregnancy.

In the early 1980s, the popularity of cocaine appeared to be growing steadily. No other drug was associated with as much glamour, notoriety, and, sadly, misinformation about its potential dangers. Even in the medical profession, cocaine was not initially thought to be highly addictive or dangerous if used intermittently. In almost every sector of society, cocaine use increased dramatically. Initially, because of its expense, cocaine was most widely used by the rich and famous. Indeed, in 1982, the most highly educated members of our society were most likely to be cocaine users. With its increasing popularity, however, production and distribution of the drug from South America increased, thus lowering the price from $150 a gram in 1980 to less than half that in most cities by 1993. The introduction of "crack" cocaine, an extremely addictive smokable form of cocaine, made initiation of cocaine use even more affordable, because crack is sold in small quantities costing from $2 to $20. Soon cocaine use was pervasive in all socioeconomic and age groups. In 1985, for example, a national survey found that 17% of American high school seniors had tried cocaine.

Gradually, evidence mounted about the hazards of using cocaine and its addictive potential. Several highly publicized incidents helped to stimulate Americans' growing awareness that cocaine use was not safe. In 1980, Richard Pryor was seriously burned while "freebasing" cocaine. Then in 1986, Len Bias, a college basketball star, died of a cocaine overdose. Efforts to educate Americans about the dangers of drug use became widespread. Groups such as the Partnership for a Drug-Free America and the Entertainment Industries Council donated time and money to produce antidrug advertisements. The media, which previously had showed cocaine to be the favorite drug of movie stars and athletes, began to show many of the same celebrities urging other Americans to stay away from cocaine.

The federal government also became more involved in fighting drug use during the 1980s. The government's "War on Drugs" has focused on reducing both the demand for cocaine and its availability on American streets. Increasing amounts of money have been spent each year; in 1991 alone, more than $10 billion was proposed to fund the federal drug strategy. Most of this money has been spent to reduce the flow of cocaine and other drugs into the United States. This effort has reduced the availability of cocaine to some degree and has probably prevented the cost of cocaine from decreasing even further. Whether this strategy has actually helped to decrease the use of cocaine is still a matter of some debate, especially when inexpensive cocaine in the form of crack is still readily available.

The medical profession has also contributed to curbing cocaine use with efforts to improve the treatment of cocaine dependence. Doctors, too, had previously been fooled into believing that cocaine was relatively harmless. Research and clinical experience, however, showed that cocaine was a powerfully addictive drug, with many serious psychological and medical effects. This experience also helped clinicians to become more skilled at treating cocaine addiction. The testing of many medications to reduce cocaine craving and the development of new psychological strategies such as cognitive and behavioral techniques to prevent cocaine relapse showed promising results. By the end of the 1980s, a growing number of cocaine-dependent people were receiving professional help for their addiction.

In the latter half of the 1980s, cocaine use in the United States declined from its peak of 5.8 million current users in 1985 to an estimated 1.9 million current users in 1991 (the National Institute on Drug Abuse defines a *current user* as someone who has used the drug within the past 30 days). Many of the factors discussed above may have contributed to this decline: increased awareness of cocaine's dangers, improvements in the treatment of cocaine addiction, and possibly decreased availability of the drug. Some epidemiologists and historians have also suggested that the cocaine epidemic may be reaching a natural and expectable end—just as many other disease epidemics are self-limited. Previous cocaine epidemics in this country, such as one in the early 20th century, also peaked after about 10 years and then declined. One must use caution, however, in comparing today's cocaine epidemic with earlier ones. In the past, cocaine was not available in as pure a form as it is now. Also, highly addictive methods of using the drug, such as smoking crack, had not been developed.

Although the statistics that showed declining cocaine use in the late 1980s were promising, there is evidence that cocaine remains a major public health problem in this country in the 1990s. Some experts believe that the growing prevalence of crack cocaine has led to a new wave of cocaine use and cocaine-related problems. Consider the following reports:

+ The number of current cocaine users actually increased to 1.9 million in 1991 from 1.6 million in 1990; much of this increase may be due to greater use of crack.
+ The number of *daily* users of cocaine continued to increase from 246,000 in 1985 to 336,000 in 1990.
+ More than 20% of babies born in some inner-city hospitals have been found to have cocaine in their bodies at birth.
+ The incidence of cocaine-related medical emergencies increased twelvefold from 1985 to 1992, with more than

30,000 emergencies recorded during a three-month period in 1992; the number of cocaine-related deaths has similarly risen.

✦ Urinalysis testing of criminal suspects in 21 major cities showed that more than 50% tested positive for cocaine in early 1990. In New York City, more than 70% of suspects had positive urine tests.

✦ Cocaine users are increasing their use of heroin to "come down" from the cocaine high. Many experts fear that a new heroin epidemic may be on the rise.

✦ Exports of cocaine to Europe doubled from 1989 to 1990; it is possible that Europe is just beginning to experience a major cocaine epidemic.

These statistics point to a disturbing trend in cocaine use: although casual use of cocaine has clearly declined, the number of daily users, in particular crack addicts, continues to climb. In addition, the extent of cocaine use by pregnant women and by people arrested for crimes is alarmingly high. Although still under study, "cocaine babies" may grow up with an array of disadvantages and disabilities (we review more thoroughly what is known about cocaine use during pregnancy in Chapter 3). There is also evidence that cocaine may increase violent behavior in some people. Although the high incidence of cocaine use in arrested suspects does not prove a causal link between cocaine use and criminal behavior, some kind of connection between cocaine use and violence appears likely. Finally, it is important that we look beyond the United States to ominous trends developing elsewhere in the world, such as in Europe. Hopefully, the gains made in awareness and treatment in the United States will help other countries prevent and fight cocaine addiction.

Why do people continue to use cocaine? What is its appeal? How does it affect the body and the mind? What can a person do if a family member or friend is using cocaine? These are some of the issues we address in this book. To gain more perspective on current cocaine use, however, we begin by looking at the place of cocaine in history.

Cocaine Use Through History

Cocaine is a naturally occurring stimulant drug found in the leaves of the coca plant, *Erythroxylon coca*. Although cocaine was not extracted from the coca leaf until the mid-19th century, archaeologists have discovered coca leaves at Peruvian grave sites dating from approximately 500 A.D., along with other items considered necessities for the afterlife. Thus, although current practices of cocaine use are relatively recent by historical standards, coca leaves have been chewed for at least 15 centuries. Coca leaves have been used in the past for a variety of religious, medicinal, and work-related reasons. They have also been the subject of a great deal of folklore over the years. Many inhabitants of coca-growing regions believed that the leaf was of divine origin, and its use was therefore reserved for members of the upper classes. One Incan myth described coca as an herb provided by the god Inti to allow the Incas to endure their difficult environmental conditions without suffering from hunger or thirst. Another myth alleged that the plant grew from the remains of a beautiful woman who had been executed for adultery, cut in half, and buried. Themes of seductiveness and danger have thus been associated with cocaine for well over a millennium.

After conquering the Incas in the 16th century, the Spanish were initially opposed to coca use because they saw worship of the drug as a barrier to religious conversion. However, the conquistadors also recognized that the leaves energized the Indians and enabled them to work long, tedious hours in gold and silver mines with little need for food or sleep. Financial considerations overcame their religious objections, and in 1569 Philip II of Spain declared the coca leaf essential to the health of the Indian. It was not long thereafter that the Spaniards began paying the Indians with coca leaves. Around this time, coca also developed a reputation as being able to treat a variety of medical disorders, including such diverse conditions as venereal diseases, headaches, asthma, rheumatism, and toothaches.

Despite the imprimatur of the Spaniards who brought coca leaves back to Europe, there was very little enthusiasm among the

Europeans for coca until 1855, when a German chemist named Friedrich Gaedecke was able to extract the active ingredient of the coca leaf, which he named *erythroxyline*. In 1859, another German, Albert Niemann, also isolated the compound and renamed it *cocaine*. This discovery sparked a flourish of experimentation with the compound, which peaked around the turn of the century. Perhaps the most notable of the drug's champions was Sigmund Freud, who performed a great deal of research on the drug, based both on personal experience and on the observation of others. In July 1884, Freud published his landmark paper entitled, "On Coca." In this work, he rhapsodized about the effects of cocaine:

> The psychic effect of cocaine consists of exhilaration and lasting euphoria, which does not differ in any way from the normal euphoria of a healthy person. . . . One senses an increase of self-control and feels more vigorous and more capable of work; on the other hand, if one works, one misses the heightening of the mental powers which alcohol, tea, or coffee induces. One is simply normal, and soon finds it difficult to believe that one is under the influence of any drug at all. . . . Long lasting intensive mental or physical work can be performed without fatigue; it is as though the need for food and sleep, which otherwise makes itself felt peremptorily at certain times of the day, were completely banished.

Freud also noted the drug's ability to relieve pain and thus paved the way for the discovery of cocaine as the first local anesthetic. He also claimed that cocaine might prove useful as a stimulant and as an aphrodisiac, as well as in the treatment of depression, gastrointestinal disturbances, wasting diseases, alcoholism, morphine addiction, and asthma. None of these predictions was supported by scientific research, however, and Freud was accused of irresponsibility by much of the scientific community because of his enthusiasm for cocaine. When Freud used the drug to treat a colleague for morphine addiction, he was dismayed to find that his patient developed a similar severe dependence on cocaine. This and other developments led Freud to eventually modify his positive feelings about cocaine.

Freud was not the only person in the late 19th century to embrace this new compound. A Corsican chemist named Angelo Mariani understood the power of this newly discovered drug, and he realized that there was money to be made from cocaine. In 1863, Mariani produced a mixture of coca leaves and wine, which he called "Vin Mariani." This tonic was phenomenally successful: among those who endorsed it were kings, queens, two popes, and such notable figures as Thomas Edison, H. G. Wells, and Jules Verne.

In 1886, an American chemist named John Styth Pemberton created a new patent medicine that was advertised as "a valuable Brain tonic and cure for all nervous affections—SICK HEADACHE, NEURALGIA, HYSTERIA, MELANCHOLY, etc." This patent medicine was later promoted as a soft drink with cocaine as its major active ingredient. Thus Coca Cola was born. Americans, as well as Europeans, were discovering around the turn of the century what South American Indians had known for hundreds of years: that the coca leaf could energize them, lift them up, and make them feel good. Although caffeine has since been substituted for cocaine as the active ingredient in Coca Cola, decocainized coca leaves are still included as part of the beverage's "natural flavors."

Cocaine use was also popularized in turn-of-the-century literature; no less a figure than Sherlock Holmes injected the drug regularly. Eventually, however, in the early part of the 20th century, this unrestrained enthusiasm for cocaine began to be tempered by increasing evidence of the drug's addictive properties. In addition, broader social factors coincided to dampen this fascination with cocaine. For example, certain "muckraking" journalists began to attack manufacturers of patent medicines because the reporters felt that the outlandish claims made for these tonics represented attempts to dupe the general public. This effort was joined by American physicians, who were becoming an increasingly organized and professional group. In addition, popular newspapers wrote about the relationship between cocaine and criminal behavior; this took a decidedly racist tone, resulting in reports of murders by "crazed (black) cocaine takers" and "attacks upon white women of the South . . . [as] the direct result of [the] coke-crazed negro brain."

7

This combination of events led to restrictions on cocaine under the Federal Harrison Narcotics Act of 1914. The Act was a paradoxical piece of legislation because it incorrectly classified cocaine as a narcotic, when in fact the drug is a stimulant. In addition, 46 of the 48 states at that time passed similar legislation to curb cocaine use, whereas only 29 states had similar laws concerning true narcotic (now termed *opioid)* drugs. From 1914 until the early 1970s, cocaine use "went underground." Use was largely confined to the fast-and-loose movie stars, jazz musicians, and wealthy thrill seekers. However, it was not used frequently by other members of the general public. Its illegal status made its price tag quite high, and a reasonable substitute in the form of amphetamine was available cheaply and legally, by prescription.

It is difficult to explain the overwhelming resurgence of cocaine use in this country beginning in the early 1970s. A number of factors, however, converged to change the drug-taking habits of America. First, an increasing segment of America had grown up using drugs. The use of marijuana and hallucinogens in the 1960s by a significant number of young Americans made many of them unafraid of the legal and potential medical consequences of so-called soft drug use. Unfortunately, cocaine had developed a reputation as being a "soft" and "safe" drug: nonaddicting, not dangerous, and short-acting: the perfect social drug. It became the drug of the rich and the powerful. Rock musicians sang its praises. Popular films portrayed cocaine as a glamorous, harmless plaything. Newspapers publicized arrests of film stars and sports celebrities who were apprehended for possession of the drug. Cocaine developed a mystique around it. Amphetamine, meanwhile, had acquired a bad reputation in the 1960s; the phrase "speed kills" had become well known among members of the drug culture. Prescriptions for amphetamine became increasingly regulated. A segment of American society was thus looking for a new stimulant drug.

At the same time, new government efforts restricted the importation of marijuana from Mexico and opioids from the Far East. As a result, drug dealers whose business in marijuana and opioids was being impeded by law enforcement efforts began diverting their focus to the cocaine trade instead.

8

The substitution of cocaine for amphetamine as the stimulant of choice in America is a rather ironic one, because a study by a group of researchers from the University of Chicago found that experienced cocaine users were unable to distinguish between the effects of cocaine and amphetamine when alternately administered both drugs intravenously without being told which was which. Other experiments have shown that cocaine users have difficulty distinguishing between cocaine and intravenous lidocaine (Xylocaine) under similar conditions. What then, are cocaine users paying for? It appears to be more than just the pharmacological effect of the drug. Cocaine use offers a sense of power and prestige that is not present with any other drug. However, this is an illusory experience, because even people with power and prestige can easily lose control of their lives as the result of using this powerful and humbling drug.

From Coca Leaf to the American Street

Despite the United States' "War on Drugs," the manufacture and distribution of cocaine remains one of the largest criminal businesses in the world. Recent United States drug strategy has emphasized two goals: reducing the supply of cocaine and reducing the demand for it. Reducing supply has involved an attempt to stop both the production and the distribution of the drug. The United States government has tried to provide incentives to farmers in Peru and other South American countries to grow crops other than coca. In addition, attempts have been made to eradicate drug syndicates at their bases; much publicity has surrounded the attempts of both Colombia and the United States to destroy the Medellin Cartel, a large drug syndicate based in Medellin, Colombia. Unfortunately, most observers estimate that this strategy has not dramatically diminished the supply of cocaine to the world. In fact, the U.S. Drug Enforcement Administration (DEA) estimates that cocaine production nearly tripled from 1988 to 1991, from 360 to 1,000 metric tons.

The Manufacture of Cocaine

The conversion of the coca leaf to the product that is illicitly marketed on the American street as "cocaine" (the quotation marks are included because the product sold on the street often contains more adulterants than pure drug) involves many steps. It begins with the coca plant itself, *Erythroxylon coca,* an evergreen shrub approximately three feet tall that grows most commonly in the eastern foothills of the Andes Mountains. More than 200 strains of coca plants have been identified. Although all contain some active alkaloids, the vast majority contain little, if any, cocaine. The bush thrives at elevations between 1,500 and 5,000 feet and generally contains a relatively small amount of active cocaine; the average Peruvian coca leaf contains approximately one-half of 1% cocaine. The bitter taste of the alkaloids probably contributes to the flourishing growth of the coca bush by making the visually attractive bush an uninviting grazing source for the local animal population.

The coca plant can be harvested between six months and three years after its first planting, depending on the strain that has been planted. Once a growing area has been established, the leaves can be harvested several times a year, simply by stripping the leaves off the bushes. The farmers then take the harvested leaves to local processing plants located in the villages, where the initial stage of extraction takes place. Here, coca paste is prepared by macerating coca leaves with kerosene, water, sodium carbonate, and sulfuric acid. Between 100 and 200 kilograms of coca leaves are necessary to produce 1 kilogram (2.2 pounds) of coca paste. The conversion of the leaf to paste thus results in an enormous reduction in bulk as well as an increasingly (40%–91%) pure product now worth four times the price of the original leaves. The decreased bulk enables drug traffickers to transport the paste far more easily than they can move massive quantities of coca leaves. Coca paste is converted into cocaine hydrochloride, the snowy white powder sold on the street, by adding a number of chemicals, which may include hydrochloric acid, potassium permanganate, acetone, ether, ammonia, calcium carbonate, sodium carbonate, sulfuric acid, and more kerosene.

Meanwhile, the price of the product has been steadily escalating. It takes approximately 2.5 kilograms of coca paste to produce a kilogram of pure cocaine hydrochloride, with a concomitant tripling of the price. In addition, the smuggling of cocaine from South America to the United States is a risky business; participants therefore expect to be well compensated for their efforts. Thus the price of cocaine is again increased by approximately 300% after it has been illegally exported to the United States. Unfortunately, the manufacture of cocaine for street distribution does not end with the smuggling of cocaine into the United States. Rather, the drug is then distributed from large drug traffickers to a series of increasingly smaller drug dealers. In each of these transactions, adulterants are added to the cocaine to make it less pure and thus more profitable to sell.

At any of these stages in distribution, cocaine hydrochloride can be converted to crack cocaine. Crack is a form of freebase cocaine that is made by dissolving powdered cocaine hydrochloride in water, adding baking soda, and heating the resultant mixture. As it cools, crystals or "rocks" form; these then can be smoked. Smaller drug dealers will often perform this simple procedure in their homes or in "rock houses" and then sell the finished product to their customers.

As cocaine use has varied in popularity, the purity of the drug sold on the streets has similarly fluctuated. In 1976, street samples submitted to drug analysis laboratories averaged 53% to 73% cocaine. Although estimates of cocaine purity in the early 1980s were considerably lower, averaging between 20% and 40%, recent reports have cited an increase in the purity of street cocaine—an ominous trend for its addictive potential. If we conservatively estimate the purity of a street sample of cocaine to be 25%, the price will have quadrupled again between importation into the United States and distribution to the user. The net price increase, then, from coca leaf to the purchase of cocaine on the street is approximately 15,000%. The current price of cocaine on the American street ranges from $50 to $100 for a gram (1/28th of an ounce). Crack is sold by the "rock" or in vials containing many pinhead-sized pieces, at a cost of $2 to $20.

The Uphill Battle Against the Cocaine Trade

Although the United States government has achieved some clear successes in its supply reduction campaign (e.g., the 1991 surrender of the reputed godfather of the Medellin syndicate to the Colombian government), the cocaine trade continues to thrive. Drug syndicates in Colombia have dispersed their smuggling and cocaine-processing operations into neighboring Latin American countries, including Brazil, Venezuela, Argentina, Ecuador, Panama, Costa Rica, Paraguay, and Chile. In addition, the DEA has estimated that a new drug syndicate based in Cali, Colombia, is currently producing 70% of the cocaine sold in the United States and 90% of cocaine reaching Europe. Robert C. Bonner, administrator of the DEA, has called the Cali syndicate "the most powerful criminal organization in the world."

The failed attempt to put drug syndicates in Colombia out of business is just one of many frustrated efforts to curb the cocaine trade. For example, as law enforcement efforts focused on eradication of local refineries in Bolivia and Peru, similar operations began in Venezuela, Panama, and Argentina. Attempts to encourage South American farmers to grow crops other than coca plants have met with extreme resistance, because it is very difficult to convince subsistence farmers and poor nations to cease growing their only profitable crop. Indeed there have been efforts in some countries to grow coca more efficiently. In the Amazon River basin of Brazil, for example, a recent strain of coca bush known as *epadu* is being cultivated. Epadu, unlike *Erythroxylon coca,* can flourish in the jungle and can grow to a height of 10 feet.

When federal drug enforcement agents began to impede drug traffic coming into Miami, traditionally the chief American port for cocaine, new smuggling routes emerged, with ports of entry in Texas, Arizona, California, and New Mexico. Currently, most cocaine smuggling occurs over the southwest borders of the United States. Government techniques to detect drugs in commercial cargo have become more and more sophisticated. Technological advances to help patrol borders have included the use of radar balloons and aircraft equipped with infrared sensors. These efforts have met with some success, as federal drug agents were able to confiscate 70 tons of cocaine in 1989 alone. At the same time, however, drug smugglers continue to improve their methods of concealing cocaine—from encasing the drug in blocks of chocolate to burying it in toxic chemicals such as powdered lye.

Although significant amounts of cocaine are seized every year, the amounts successfully entering the United States are nevertheless much higher. It is estimated that U.S. Customs can check less than 5% of the shipping containers that enter American ports annually. American borders are thousands of miles long, and no amount of sophisticated detection equipment can successfully patrol every mile. Meanwhile, cocaine production continues to increase, with an estimated supply of 1,000 metric tons in 1991. Large drug busts may decrease the supply of cocaine temporarily, resulting in increased wholesale prices; however, in recent years, these wholesale price increases have not necessarily resulted in increased street prices, because dealers often compensate by adding more adulterants to the cocaine they buy, thus extending the value while decreasing the purity.

The Social Costs of Cocaine Use

Once the cocaine is in the United States, its distribution and sale comprises another huge business. Typically, each major city is dominated by one or more criminal organization that controls cocaine selling throughout the city. In some cities, such as Los Angeles, pre-existing gangs have taken on much of the distribution and sale of cocaine. In the mid-1980s, highly organized Jamaican gangs became involved in crack dealing in Miami and New York. These so-called posses were known for their extraordinary violence and mobility; gang members moved to cities throughout the country, starting up new crack businesses. Today, it is estimated that approximately 40 of these posses exist, with a membership of 22,000, controlling one-third of the crack trade in America. Although the leaders of these drug-dealing organizations can make hundreds of thousands of dollars a year, the street-level dealers who work for them sometimes make barely enough money to survive and support their own drug addictions. A recent study by the Rand Corporation found that street dealers stood a 1-in-70 chance of getting killed, a 1-in-14 chance of severe injury, and a 2-in-9 chance of going to jail. Despite these odds, many inner-city youths are still attracted to drug-dealing and the prospect of rising through the ranks to make "crazy money."

Drug dealing and drug use in the United States have brought with them a scourge of crime and violence. The Federal Bureau of Investigation estimates that there are more than one million arrests each year for drug abuse violations. Violent crime continues to rise in the United States, with rates for 1990 up 10% from the year before; much of this crime is thought to be drug related. Ironically, as overall use of cocaine declines, street dealers fight over fewer customers, resulting in more drug-related shootings, stabbings, and assaults. Given the serious repercussions of cocaine use in this country, it is clear that curbing addiction to the drug will remain a major public health and policy challenge during the 1990s.

Chapter 2

How Cocaine Is Used

Intranasal Cocaine Use ("Snorting")

Although increasing numbers of people addicted to cocaine are smoking "crack" or using cocaine intravenously, intranasal use ("snorting") remains a common method of use in the United States. In particular, many individuals often prefer to use the drug intranasally when first using cocaine. Progression to smoking crack or to using cocaine intravenously, to get a faster and more intense "high," can occur as a person's dependence on cocaine becomes more severe. Surveys from the 1-800-COCAINE telephone help-line, for example, have revealed that the percentage of callers reporting intranasal use declined from 61% in 1983 to 39% by 1989. At the same time, of all callers, those reporting crack use increased from 21% to 55%. Most of these individuals reported switching to crack after trying intranasal cocaine.

To use cocaine intranasally, crystalline cocaine hydrochloride purchased on the street is placed on a flat shiny surface—typically, a mirror, glass coffee table, or piece of marble. The cocaine is then chopped finely with a razor blade and arranged into thin lines about an eighth of an inch wide and one or two inches long. About 20 to 40 lines can be made from one gram of cocaine, which is purchased on the street for $50 to $100. A line of cocaine is inhaled, often with great ceremony, through a straw, a rolled-up dollar bill, or a thin cylindrical object called a "tooter." The drug's effects typically begin 30 seconds to 2 minutes after snorting and peak within 10 to 20 minutes. After 45 to 60 minutes, the effects begin to wear off.

The amount of active drug in a line of cocaine varies, depending on the amount of adulterant that has been added. If the drug is only 10% pure, one line will contain only about 3 milligrams of active drug. If, on the other hand, the cocaine is 50% pure, a line may contain approximately 15 milligrams of active drug. These figures assume importance because research has shown that volunteers given less than 10 milligrams of pure cocaine intranasally are unable to distinguish the effects of the drug from a placebo. Because street cocaine is sometimes so impure that a line may contain less than 10 milligrams of active drug, the pharmacological effect from such a preparation should be negligible. However, many drug users continue to get high from an amount of drug that has been shown in scientific experiments to be no more powerful than an inactive white powder. Thus there must be more factors involved in the cocaine intoxication than the direct chemical effect.

It is a well-known phenomenon among researchers and drug users that a person's experience while on a drug is strongly affected by the setting in which he or she uses the drug and the expectations he or she has of the drug's effects. For example, if someone anticipates becoming intoxicated, he or she is more likely to feel high after using a drug than is someone who expects to feel nothing. Getting high is thus, in part, a learned experience: one learns how to act, how to feel, and what sensations to anticipate and guard against. This phenomenon was illustrated clearly in a fascinating study of marijuana smokers by Dr. Reese Jones at the University of California, San Francisco. In this study, many individuals who unknowingly smoked marijuana cigarettes with little or no tetrahydrocannabinol (THC; the psychoactive ingredient in marijuana) claimed to feel intoxicated when they thought they were smoking bona fide marijuana.

Effects of Intranasal Use

After inhalation, cocaine is rapidly absorbed into the bloodstream—first into the small blood vessels of the nose and then into the general circulation. The drug can be detected in the blood within three minutes after use, and the amount of drug in the blood (the blood level) increases quickly, peaking between 15 minutes and an hour after the drug has been taken. Studies show that there is a good correlation between blood levels of cocaine and its physiological and psychological effects.

The effects of cocaine on mood are most prominent 15 to 30 minutes after intranasal administration. Cardiovascular changes, including an increased heart rate and blood pressure, occur most strongly in 15 to 20 minutes. Although the emotional and cardiovascular effects of cocaine wear off approximately an hour after intranasal use, the drug remains in the bloodstream for four to six hours. One reason that cocaine may remain in the body so long is its ability to constrict the blood vessels in the nose, thus retarding the absorption of the drug into the general circulation. Indeed, cocaine can be detected in the nose for up to three hours after drug use. The discrepancy between the drug's brief duration of action and its prolonged presence in the blood may also be explained by the theory that cocaine makes people euphoric only as the amount of drug in the blood is rising. When the blood level plateaus and decreases, the drug may have little effect. In some cases, users with falling blood levels may feel as if they are coming off of the drug.

Although some people who use cocaine experience few untoward effects after occasional use, other individuals feel anxious, depressed, tired, and irritable approximately an hour after snorting small amounts of the drug. These symptoms may be accompanied by a desire for more cocaine. Although it is not known how many people in the general population have the latter response to cocaine use, a study by Dr. Richard Resnick and his colleagues at New York Medical College found that a subgroup of experienced cocaine users who volunteered for a study on the effects of cocaine experienced this "crash" or "postcoke blues" after taking 25 milligrams (approximately two lines) of cocaine intranasally. In these and other vulnerable individuals, a combination of postcocaine depression, drug craving, and drug availability may lead to repetitive use and, in some cases, cocaine dependence.

Medical Complications of Intranasal Use

Physical symptoms frequently experienced by intranasal cocaine users include nasal congestion and cold symptoms. In severe cases, they may suffer from ulceration of nasal tissue and, less often, perforation of the nasal septum (the hard portion of the nose between the two nostrils). Some individuals attempt to avert these difficulties by cleaning their noses with a saltwater solution or by using glycerin, vitamin E, or petroleum jelly (Vaseline). These home remedies and prophylactic measures are generally unsuccessful if cocaine use continues. Frequent use of nasal decongestants, particularly nasal sprays, is also common among intranasal cocaine users. Some individuals can become dependent on these sprays and may experience a worsening of their symptoms when they try to discontinue these over-the-counter preparations. Specialized medical treatment may be necessary to wean such individuals from their nasal sprays.

The patterns of use among intranasal users vary widely. Whereas intravenous injection of cocaine generally implies heavy involvement with the drug, intranasal use may be seen in those who try the drug once out of curiosity, as well as in addicts who spend more than $1,000 a week on the drug. Many people have gathered the impression that "only snorting" cocaine is safe and that it is very difficult to become addicted to cocaine via this "harmless" route of administration, but this idea has been clearly shown to be untrue. Although snorting cocaine may be less addicting than smoking crack or injecting cocaine intravenously, this does not in any way make it safe. For example, many of the cocaine-dependent patients admitted to our treatment facility have been exclusively intranasal users and have experienced the same serious consequences of cocaine use as those who smoke or inject it. Thus "merely" snorting cocaine offers no protection against the serious consequences of the drug.

Smoking Cocaine

Smoking crack cocaine has become very popular since its introduction in the United States in 1985. Indeed, the National Institute on Drug Abuse 1991 Household Survey reported that crack was used by approximately one million of the six million individuals who used cocaine at least once during that year. Among the 625,000 individuals who used cocaine at least once a week, the proportion of crack users was likely much higher. Epidemiological studies show that crack is most widely used by young adults, typically men, who are heavy users of other drugs. A Canadian study by Dr. Reginald Smart showed that crack users are typically younger than intranasal users (with an average age of 14 years) and are more likely to also use other drugs, such as phencyclidine (PCP), tranquilizers, heroin, stimulants, and glue. In Miami, 96% of street youths involved in crime report that they have used crack at some time.

Some inpatient detoxification units have been designated as specialized "crack units" in response to increased admissions of crack addicts. One such unit in Brooklyn was studied by Dr. Barbara Wallace, who found that crack users were largely unemployed, poorly educated individuals, many of whom had been exposed to domestic violence and alcoholism. Moreover, 39% of these individuals met criteria for major depression or dysthymia.

Before crack became widespread in the United States, cocaine smoking in the form of coca paste (see below) was popular in South America. Although coca paste smoking never took hold in the United States, smoking cocaine freebase (see below) appeared in the United States as early as 1974. Crack is cocaine freebase sold in a ready-to-smoke form. The success of crack has been largely attributed to a successful marketing campaign by drug dealers and traffickers. A simple production technique created a packaged, ready-to-use product with a low unit price that gives an intense, almost instantaneous high. Given these characteristics, it is not surprising that crack is so widely used. Before looking more closely at crack and how it is used, however, we will first turn our attention to its predecessor, coca paste.

Coca Paste

The practice of smoking coca paste first received attention in the early 1970s, when Peruvian doctors began to see an increasing number of young people who were experiencing severe physical and psychological difficulties as a result of repetitive smoking. Many of these individuals were hospitalized because of compulsive use of the drug, whereas others died as the result of acute cocaine intoxication.

Coca paste consists of a mixture of cocaine, kerosene, sulfuric acid, and sodium carbonate. The purity of the paste may vary widely; laboratory analyses have revealed concentrations of cocaine ranging from 40% to 91%. The white or brown paste is allowed to dry after being manufactured; it is then placed at the end of a tobacco or marijuana cigarette, ignited, and inhaled deeply.

Coca paste is absorbed into the blood very rapidly after smoking; studies of healthy volunteers have shown that the blood level of cocaine after smoking paste rises as rapidly as after intravenous injection of the drug. Physical effects include increased pulse, blood pressure, respiratory rate, and body temperature. Dilated pupils, muscle tension, tremulousness, and heavy perspiration are also common effects of the drug. Although initial use of the drug is characterized by euphoria, gregariousness, and a sense of well-being, repeated exposure frequently causes anxiety, hostility, and extreme depression. As people smoke more heavily, the period of euphoria may last for only a few seconds, followed by anxiety and a craving for more cocaine. Long-term users may also drink alcohol to decrease their anxiety and alter the rapidly changing moods caused by coca paste.

Further use of coca paste can lead to a wide variety of symptoms: numbness in the mouth, a burning sensation in the eyes, pounding heartbeat, tremulous limbs, headache, insomnia, dizziness, abdominal pain, and profuse sweating. Continued use may lead to visual and auditory misperceptions, as harmless objects and noises may begin to appear threatening. Feelings of anxiety may become overwhelming and are sometimes accompanied by aggressiveness or severe depression. Hallucinations may occur if the drug use continues; the long-term smoker may hear, see, feel, or smell things that are not there, and he or she may become frankly paranoid. Individuals continuing to smoke the drug may develop "coca paste psychosis," characterized by extreme hypervigilance, paranoid delusions, and hallucinations. This is an extremely serious condition in which overdoses, suicides, and homicides have occurred. Unfortunately, attempts to treat compulsive coca paste smoking in South America have often been unsuccessful; relapse rates are high and the consequences of ongoing coca paste smoking can be grave.

Smoking Crack (Cocaine Freebase)

Crack is produced by combining cocaine hydrochloride with water and sodium bicarbonate (baking soda). This mixture is heated until all the water has evaporated. The resultant product is small chips, consisting of the alkaline precipitate of cocaine. These white "rocks," which have the texture of porcelain, are ready to smoke; they may contain in excess of 75% pure cocaine and are often sold for as little as $2 to $20 each. The low price, ease of use, high purity, and extremely addictive nature of crack (so named because of the cracking sound sometimes made during the vaporization process) explain its rapid spread among cocaine users in the United States.

In the 1970s and early 1980s, freebase was often prepared by adding ammonia, rather than baking soda, to cocaine hydrochloride; ether was frequently added to extract the cocaine base. Because preparing and using cocaine freebase in this manner involved volatile chemicals such as ether and the use of high heat (often from acetylene or butane torches), the process was quite dangerous. Indeed, comedian Richard Pryor was seriously burned when he set himself on fire while freebasing. The elimination of these steps in preparing crack also helps to account for its popularity.

Although, like coca paste, crack can be added to a tobacco or marijuana cigarette, it is usually placed in a pipe. The drug is then ignited and deeply inhaled, as in marijuana and coca paste smoking. Inhalation from a pipe is typically accompanied by the loss of a great deal of cocaine. In fact, some studies have shown that only 1% to 5% of the initial cocaine is actually inhaled by this method. Smoking crack through a cigarette is similarly inefficient; nearly half of the cocaine is lost through the burning end of the cigarette, and only about 6% is inhaled.

21

Crack smoking causes a very rapid rise in the blood level of cocaine and produces almost instantaneous psychological effects, which peak in about five minutes. The user experiences intense euphoria almost immediately after inhalation, accompanied by a rise in blood pressure, pulse, body temperature, and respiratory rate. A research study conducted by Dr. Mario Perez-Reyes at the University of North Carolina revealed that the psychological and physical effects of smoking cocaine were as powerful as those produced by an injection of intravenous cocaine. The euphoria produced by smoking is quite short lived, however, ending 10 to 20 minutes after inhalation. Although some crack smokers experience little in the way of aftereffects, many become quite anxious and depressed after the drug has worn off; these feelings are sometimes accompanied by severe drug craving. Indeed, Dr. Perez-Reyes found that cocaine smokers reported a higher degree of craving for cocaine after drug use than did intravenous users.

Some of the characteristics of crack that make it so addictive include the intensity of euphoria it produces, its nearly immediate onset of action, and the brevity of the high. In addition, the aftermath of crack use is often characterized by severe craving for more drug. Although some individuals may stop after limiting themselves to one or two "hits," repetitive use is a more common pattern. Because the psychological effects of smoking cocaine peak five minutes after use, only to be followed by severe depression, agitation, and drug craving ("crashing") 10 minutes later, many users try to ward off these symptoms by smoking again before they occur. Because the period of time between intoxication and crashing is so short, these individuals may end up smoking cocaine almost continuously, remaining in a nearly constant state of intoxication until the drug supply has been exhausted. This pattern of cocaine use is called a "run," and may last from several hours to a number of days.

Many of the symptoms produced by long-term crack smoking are similar to those described above for coca paste smoking. In addition, other hazards have been reported. Long-term crack smoking may cause a form of lung disease that has been termed *crack lung* (see Chapter 3). Moreover, smoking crack has been reported to produce burns of the larynx.

Just as drug paraphernalia is an important aspect of cocaine use, the location where crack is used can take on similar importance. This may explain the prevalence of "crack houses," also known as "rock houses" or "base houses." A crack house is a house or apartment where customers come to buy and use crack cocaine. In New York City alone it is estimated that hundreds of these houses exist, in abandoned buildings, apartments, and brownstones. A customer usually pays a nominal fee to enter, and private rooms may be available for an hourly rate. Customers often bring their own drug paraphernalia, such as pipes, but a stove is often available for those who want to convert powdered cocaine into crack. When a customer runs out of cocaine, there is usually someone at the house who will leave to buy more cocaine, in exchange for a tip and a share of the drugs. In some houses, sex is exchanged for drugs.

Intravenous Cocaine Use

Perhaps the most perilous method of cocaine administration is intravenous use. In addition to its high addiction liability (much like cocaine smoking), intravenous use carries with it the additional hazard of unsterile needles. Intravenous use is a more common method of administration among people addicted to cocaine than among occasional users. Because taking poor care of oneself is frequently part of the addictive process, many individuals with severe cocaine dependence share needles and expose themselves to serious medical complications, in particular hepatitis, endocarditis, and acquired immunodeficiency syndrome (AIDS). (These diseases are discussed in Chapter 3.)

Cocaine is prepared for intravenous administration by placing between one-tenth and one-quarter of a gram in a spoon and then adding water. This aqueous solution is then strained, after which it is drawn up into a syringe and injected into a vein. Euphoria occurs almost immediately.

With more frequent use, some individuals gradually increase their dosage of cocaine, so that they may inject up to a gram at a time. Like cocaine smokers, intravenous users frequently take cocaine in sprees ("runs"): discrete episodes of highly intensive drug use. During these periods, they may use massive amounts of cocaine, perhaps spending thousands of dollars in a week. A study by Drs. Frank Gawin and Herbert Kleber showed that although intravenous and intranasal cocaine users both took similar amounts of cocaine when averaged out over a week, the intravenous users tended to use very large amounts of cocaine in discrete, brief periods, whereas the intranasal users took the drug more often but in lower doses. Cocaine smokers in their study used almost twice as much cocaine as that used by the other two groups, with longer runs and even heavier drug use than the intravenous users.

Intravenous use of cocaine is highly addictive for the same reasons that freebase or crack smoking is: the intensity of the euphoria, the nearly immediate onset of action, and the brevity of the high. An intravenous user may become depressed and irritable within 5 to 15 minutes after drug use. This "crash" frequently leads to frantic repeated injections, sometimes occurring as often as every 5 minutes. This scenario was described by one patient, as follows:

> Once I started shooting coke, my life became a complete nightmare. It was as if I was a slave to the needle. Within literally a couple of minutes after sticking the needle into my arm, I was a basket case. I would stand around sweating and shaking, and I'd be paranoid that the police were going to break into my house. The worst part was that in spite of all this, I couldn't wait to "boot" [inject] more coke. That needle became my entire world. By the end of a run, I'd be stabbing myself all over the place looking for a vein, getting sloppier each time. There would be blood dripping all over the floor, all over my clothes, all over everything, and I didn't care at all.

A particularly dangerous phenomenon among intravenous cocaine users is "speedballing," which involves injecting cocaine and heroin together. The purpose of this practice is to buffer ("mellow out") the stimulant effects of cocaine with the more sedating, relaxing effects of heroin. In addition, the longer-lasting opiate effect helps to guard against the depression that frequently follows cocaine use. Some users believe that the combination of an "upper" (cocaine) and a "downer" (heroin) makes the combination safer than either of the two drugs taken individually. This presumption is untrue; the potentially fatal respiratory depression caused by heroin may be made more severe by cocaine, thus rendering the combination of cocaine and heroin even more dangerous than the use of either drug alone.

As we discuss in Chapter 3, one of the major hazards of intravenous cocaine use is the risk involved in using unsterile needles. Insulin syringes (legally sold by prescription only) are typically sold on the street for approximately $3 each, although the price can go much higher in some areas. However, as for any other commodity, the price is dictated in part by the quality of the product. Thus used needles are sold more cheaply than new, sterile needles. The most desperate addicts and those with the fewest financial resources are thus most likely to use contaminated needles. They therefore carry a higher risk of acquiring and spreading needle-related infections.

Chapter 3

The Effects of Cocaine on the Body

In discussing the effects of cocaine on the body, it is important to keep in mind that street preparations of cocaine have been adulterated with a variety of "cuts" (see Table 1), all of which are designed to dilute the amount of pure cocaine being sold and thus increase the profit to the seller. Because the product advertised as "cocaine" may contain as little as 10% pure drug, the potential physical problems resulting from street cocaine will depend in part on the specific cuts being used.

Cocaine can be taken into the body intranasally, intravenously, orally, by smoking, or through other mucous membranes including the vagina, gums, or urethra. Once inside the body, cocaine is taken up by a large number of body organs, including the liver, kidney, heart, and brain; some of the drug also penetrates into fat tissue. The blood level of cocaine is highest approximately five minutes after smoking or taking the drug intravenously; peak blood levels tend to occur 15 to 60 minutes after snorting.

Cocaine is broken down quickly by the body into inactive by-products and for the most part is eliminated within 24 hours. The drug appears to be broken down largely by an enzyme in the blood called *pseudocholinesterase*. This information is important because a small number of people are born with a deficiency of this enzyme. This deficiency would not otherwise be detected except through the administration of certain general anesthetics that are also broken down by the same enzyme. Thus an individual with a pseudocholinesterase deficiency might have a severe toxic or even fatal reaction to even a small amount of cocaine, as the ordinarily rapid

Table 1.   Common adulterants ("cuts") used to dilute cocaine

Sugars	Miscellaneous fillers
Lactose	Cornstarch
Glucose	Flour
Mannitol	Talc
Inositol	Phencyclidine (PCP)
Other local anesthetics	Heroin
Lidocaine	Quinine
Tetracaine	
Procaine	
Benzocaine	

breakdown of the drug cannot occur. Cocaine is metabolized into a number of by-products, some of them active and others inactive. The by-product most commonly detected in people's urine is *benzoylecgonine*; this metabolite can be detected for up to several days after cocaine use.

General Physical Effects of Cocaine

The major medical use for cocaine today is as a local anesthetic in ear, nose, and throat surgery. Cocaine was, in fact, the first local anesthetic, having initially been used in eye surgery a century ago. The reason cocaine is still preferred as a local anesthetic in some surgical procedures is its ability to constrict blood vessels in the area to which it has been applied. This "vasoconstrictor" effect decreases bleeding during surgery, thus allowing the surgeon to see the operative field more clearly. Because the ear, nose, and throat contain many blood vessels, cocaine is a particularly valuable anesthetic in this type of surgery. We discuss later how cocaine-induced vasoconstriction can also cause serious medical problems when the drug is used repeatedly or in large doses.

Another major effect of cocaine is its activation of the sympathetic nervous system, which controls numerous functions of the brain and other organs, including blood pressure, heart rate, contractility of heart muscle, blood sugar level, mood, and appetite. The sympathetic nervous system is the part of the body that, among other functions, controls the "fight or flight" response. When a person experiences danger or other significant stress, the sympathetic nervous system can respond by triggering the release of certain hormones (predominantly epinephrine) and neurotransmitters (e.g., norepinephrine and dopamine) that help the body respond to the danger. When the sympathetic nervous system is activated, the heart pumps faster and more powerfully to increase the flow of blood into critical areas. Blood pressure rises, body temperature increases, and the individual becomes more activated and alert. The need for food and sleep diminishes, because (in an evolutionary sense) these activities only interfere with the need to fight or run. By activating the sympathetic nervous system, cocaine causes euphoria, decreased appetite, mental stimulation, rapid heartbeat, increased blood pressure, elevated body temperature, an increased rate of breathing, more rapid brain electrical activity, and an elevated blood sugar level. Although some of these effects are generally sought out by cocaine users, an excess of these physiological responses can precipitate significant problems.

Medical Complications From Cocaine Use

The incidence of adverse medical effects from using cocaine appears to have reached an all-time high. The number of cocaine-related emergencies as recorded by the federal government's Drug Abuse Warning Network increased by 30% from 1990 to 1991, with more than 25,000 cocaine-related emergencies reported in a three-month period during 1991. Cocaine-related deaths have also been increasing; in 1989, almost 2,500 people died from cocaine overdose. In addition to fatal overdose, many other medical complications can occur as a consequence of cocaine use. These adverse effects can be divided into several major categories (see Table 2). First, complications may occur immediately as the result of taking too much cocaine, that is, an overdose. Second, there are long-term effects that occur as the result of repeated cocaine use. In addition to the direct results of the drug, medical complications in cocaine users may be caused by paraphernalia (in particular, unsterile needles) or adulterants ("cuts"). Finally, long-term cocaine users frequently develop psychiatric problems and engage in a lifestyle that may increase their risk to develop certain medical complications.

A recent study by Dr. Steven Brody and co-workers in Atlanta reviewed all of the cocaine-related medical problems seen in their emergency room over a six-month period. Almost 50% of the 233 study patients used cocaine intravenously, whereas another 23% smoked cocaine, suggesting that individuals using cocaine by these routes of administration may experience the greatest risk of adverse physical effects. Forty percent of the patients studied went to the emergency room because they were experiencing chest pain. Other frequent complaints were (in order of decreasing frequency) shortness of breath, anxiety, and heart palpitations. Although many of these cocaine-related emergency room visits did not turn out to be serious, 10% of these individuals required hospital admission, and 1% died.

Cocaine Overdose—
How Cocaine Can Kill

The lethal effects of cocaine represent an exaggeration of the typical physical effects produced by the drug. Thus there are many mechanisms by which cocaine can cause a fatal overdose. All of the potentially fatal effects below have been seen in individuals who use intranasally and intravenously, as well as those who smoke cocaine. Using cocaine intranasally does not prevent cocaine overdose.

1. Cocaine use can cause a myocardial infarction (i.e., a heart attack). Heart attacks occur when the heart muscle does not receive enough oxygen and is therefore unable to keep pumping

blood to the rest of the body. The cardinal symptoms of a heart attack are chest pain and, sometimes, shortness of breath. However, having chest pain does not necessarily mean that an individual is having a heart attack. Heart attacks can be caused by increased heart rate and arrhythmias (discussed further below),

Table 2. Medical complications from cocaine use

I. Generalized drug effects
   A. Overdose
      1. Heart attack
      2. Rapid irregular heartbeat (ventricular tachycardia or fibrillation)
      3. Cerebral hemorrhage
      4. Heatstroke
      5. Seizures
      6. Respiratory failure
   B. Chronic nasal problems
   C. Lung damage from smoking cocaine
   D. Heart damage (cardiomyopathy)
   E. Vitamin deficiencies
   F. Sexual difficulties

II. Complications during pregnancy associated with cocaine use
   A. Premature birth
   B. Low birth weight
   C. Fetal abnormalities

III. Complications due to using unsterile needles
   A. Skin infections
   B. Hepatitis
   C. Endocarditis
   D. Acquired immunodeficiency syndrome (AIDS)

IV. Complications due to adulterants ("cuts")
   A. Inflammation in lungs
   B. Virtually anything, depending on the adulterant

V. Complications due to psychiatric effects and life-style
   A. Polysubstance abuse
   B. Suicide
   C. Accidents
   D. Homicide

increased blood pressure, increased demand for oxygen by the heart, or a narrowing or spasm of the blood vessels that supply oxygen to the heart (the coronary arteries). Cocaine can cause all of these adverse effects. An individual does not have to have preexisting heart disease or coronary artery disease to have a heart attack after using cocaine.

2. Cocaine increases heart rate. If a person's heart beats too rapidly, the steady rhythm of the heart may be disturbed, and irregular electrical activity may occur. Indeed, feeling their heart "skipping a beat" is one of the most common reactions that cocaine users experience. Abnormal heart rhythm may be quite dangerous in certain individuals and may quickly lead to a dangerous heart irregularity known as *ventricular tachycardia* (extremely rapid, although regular, contraction of the heart) or to *ventricular fibrillation* (irregular and very weak motions of the heart); either of these conditions can be quickly fatal.

3. The ability of cocaine to increase blood pressure can also cause trouble; if a person's blood pressure increases too rapidly or too much, a weak-walled blood vessel in the brain may burst under increased pressure, causing a cerebral hemorrhage (bleeding into the brain). A cerebral hemorrhage is often fatal.

4. The increased body temperature that cocaine causes may occasionally reach dangerous heights in certain individuals; this complication is known as *hyperpyrexia*.

5. Cocaine use, sometimes at relatively low doses, can precipitate grand mal seizures (epileptic convulsions). Indeed, long-term cocaine use may eventually sensitize the individual to further seizures at increasingly lower doses, a phenomenon known medically as *kindling*. Although grand mal seizures are not in themselves always life-threatening, they may be fatal under some circumstances. For example, several seizures may occur rapidly in succession, a very serious and sometimes fatal condition known as *status epilepticus*. A seizure may also occur at an inopportune moment, such as while driving a car or crossing the street. Clearly, fatalities can also occur at these times.

6. Respiratory difficulties are another cause of cocaine-related deaths. As users increase their dose of cocaine, the deep rapid

respirations that often occur after low-to-moderate doses may give way to labored breathing; an overdose may produce gasping: shallow irregular breaths that can culminate in respiratory arrest (cessation of breathing). Respiratory symptoms can occur in all cocaine users, regardless of the way in which cocaine is used. Certain lung problems that are specific to users who smoke cocaine are discussed later in this chapter.

7. Cocaine overdoses may also occur in special populations. We have already mentioned the rare individuals who are born with a deficiency of pseudocholinesterase, an enzyme that breaks down cocaine. Deaths have been reported in such individuals who have been given as little as 20 milligrams of cocaine as a local anesthetic. Cocaine may also increase levels of blood sugar, thus harming patients with diabetes. Individuals with angina pectoris (chest pain due to coronary artery disease) may also aggravate their condition through cocaine use.

Some people want to know a "safe" way to use cocaine. Unfortunately, there is no clear answer to this. Because individuals vary in their sensitivity to the drug, a dose that may be "safe" in one person may precipitate severe medical difficulties or even death in another. For example, people with pseudocholinesterase deficiency can have severe reactions to even minute doses of cocaine. It is therefore reasonable to conclude that there is no predictably safe dose of cocaine.

Effects of Long-Term Cocaine Use

The medical complications that may occur as the result of repeated cocaine use can be divided into several major categories. First is the group of complications that occur because of the repeated use of cocaine itself. The other medical problems develop as the result of the adulterants (cuts), drug paraphernalia (e.g., unsterile needles), psychiatric symptoms, or life-styles that generally accompany cocaine use.

Medical Complications Due to Effects of Cocaine Itself

Nose Problems

The area most often damaged by intranasal cocaine use is the site where cocaine enters the body—the nose. As mentioned before, cocaine is a very powerful vasoconstrictor; thus blood vessels in the area exposed to cocaine are reduced in size, and blood flow to that area is diminished. Because blood transports oxygen and other nutrients required to keep body tissues alive and healthy, an area that is repeatedly exposed to cocaine will, in essence, be malnourished. Thus the mucous membranes of the nose may become irritated and inflamed, and painful ulcers may develop inside the nostrils. Chronic sneezing, frequent nosebleeds, and nasal congestion are common symptoms. Experienced cocaine users frequently try to avert these consequences by rinsing their nasal passages with salt water or by applying glycerin, vitamin E, or petroleum jelly (Vaseline) to their noses. However, these home remedies are generally unsuccessful, and they are frequently applied less often as cocaine use increases. Long-term intranasal cocaine use can sometimes lead to tissue death and eventual perforation of the nasal septum (the portion of the nose that separates the two nostrils); the only treatment for this condition is plastic surgery.

Heart Problems

In addition to causing heart attacks and abnormal heart rhythms, long-term cocaine use can damage the heart muscle and therefore prevent it from contracting normally. This condition is known as *cardiomyopathy.* Cardiomyopathy may be caused by a direct toxic effect of cocaine on the heart. People who have cardiomyopathy are more susceptible to having heart attacks and to sudden cardiac death.

Lung Problems

Respiratory arrest from a fatal overdose of cocaine may occur regardless of the way in which cocaine is used. There are some lung problems, however, that are specifically caused by smoking cocaine. The lungs of freebase smokers frequently show a decreased ability to perform one of their major tasks: the transportation of oxygen into the blood. It has been hypothesized that the vasoconstrictor effect of cocaine, which causes so much obvious damage in the nostrils of intranasal users, may impair pulmonary (lung) function by causing similar changes in the blood vessels of the lungs. Additionally, an acute pulmonary syndrome known as *crack lung* can occur in cocaine smokers. Patients with this syndrome may experience chest pain, shortness of breath, or coughing up blood. Symptoms may begin almost immediately after smoking crack, or up to 48 hours after crack was last used. In general, this syndrome resolves spontaneously, but some people require medications or sometimes mechanical ventilation to recover.

Vitamin Deficiencies

One of the prominent effects of cocaine is its ability to suppress appetite and cause weight loss. For many users, this property is highly desirable. Frequently accompanying the weight loss, however, is a deficiency of vitamins, particularly the water-soluble B and C vitamins. Indeed, in an early study, Dr. Mark Gold reported that 19 of 26 cocaine users hospitalized at Fair Oaks Hospital in Summit, New Jersey, were deficient in at least one vitamin, with vitamin B6 (pyridoxine) deficiency being most common. In addition to causing vitamin deficiencies, the weight loss that often accompanies long-term cocaine use may result in other manifestations of malnutrition, including anemia and metabolic abnormalities.

Seizures (Convulsions)

One of the most dangerous complications of cocaine use is grand mal seizures, such as those that occur in people who have epilepsy.

Seizures occur as a result of the uncontrolled release of electrical discharges in the brain. Because cocaine reduces the threshold for seizures, vulnerable individuals may suffer a convulsion after just a single dose of cocaine. For others, repeated use of cocaine may gradually lower the seizure threshold. This kindling effect may eventually lead to the development of seizures, which can be extremely dangerous and are sometimes fatal.

Sexual Difficulties

One frequently cited reason for cocaine use is its reputation as an aphrodisiac. This perception was not confirmed, however, in a study of regular cocaine users by University of California, Los Angeles, psychologist Ronald Siegel; he found that only 13% of those surveyed claimed to experience increased sexual stimulation from cocaine use. Although the mental stimulation and disinhibition from cocaine may initially heighten sexual pleasure, higher doses and more frequent drug use generally lead to sexual dysfunction. Impotence and inability to ejaculate are common complaints in male cocaine users; decreased desire for sex becomes the norm in users of both sexes. Some people who initially find sex more pleasurable while intoxicated may become dependent on the use of cocaine for sexual arousal; they may even find themselves unable to enjoy sex at all for a long period of time following long-term cocaine use. Some cocaine users attempt to increase their sexual pleasure by directly applying the drug to their genitals. Because cocaine is a local anesthetic, placing it on a mucous membrane such as the penis or clitoris may in fact decrease sensation and prolong sexual intercourse. Unfortunately, this practice can be quite hazardous, because the tissues to which cocaine has been applied may receive decreased blood flow and may dry up and become ulcerated.

Adverse Effects of Cocaine on Pregnancy

There has been much focus recently on cocaine use during pregnancy, with growing concern about adverse effects on children exposed to cocaine in utero. In fact, the degree of fetal damage caused by cocaine itself is still controversial, mainly because it is difficult to isolate the effects of cocaine from the effects of other dangers to which cocaine-using pregnant women are frequently exposed. Until further studies can clarify this issue, however, it is safest to assume that cocaine use during pregnancy is dangerous.

Cocaine use during pregnancy has tragically become relatively common—a fact that has mobilized health personnel, educators, and even the criminal justice system to try to find solutions to this problem. The National Association for Perinatal Addiction Research and Education (NAPARE) estimates that 1 out of 10 newborns is exposed to one or more illicit drugs in utero—with the most common drug being cocaine. Moreover, a recent large-scale drug screening study in an urban obstetric population found that 31% of the newborns tested positive for cocaine in their bodies.

In addition to the immeasurable cost of damaged lives is the ever-growing financial burden this problem is creating. A recent study in Florida estimated that the hospital costs for cocaine-exposed infants were more than twice as high per patient as for other infants. Other costs are also adding up. For example, in New York City, foster home placements of drug-exposed babies cost $795 million dollars a year. Future costs, including special education for these children, has yet to be calculated.

Cocaine potentially affects the fetus in many ways. Cocaine is highly fat soluble, and thus passes easily into the placenta, which provides nourishment for the fetus. Cocaine has been shown to cause vasoconstriction and increased heart rate in the fetus just as it does in the actual user of the drug. This vasoconstriction can lead to decreased oxygen supply to the fetus as it is developing. Decreased oxygen supply could result in growth retardation or fetal disruption, causing premature birth. Cocaine has also been shown to stimulate the pregnant uterus to contract, thus perhaps precipitating premature birth. Finally, cocaine may exert direct toxicity on the developing fetal central nervous system. As reviewed in Chapter 4, cocaine has direct effects on chemicals in the brain, such as dopamine and norepinephrine, which are important in normal brain functioning. Disruption of these neurochemicals in the fetus, especially during the first trimester when the fetal nervous system is still being formed, may lead to neurological and behavioral difficulties after birth.

Much research has been conducted to try to establish a link between cocaine use during pregnancy and fetal abnormalities or neurobehavioral difficulties after birth. These studies have shown that a multitude of complications can occur in women who use cocaine during pregnancy. Adverse effects that have been reported in children exposed to cocaine in utero include premature birth, low birth weight, decreased head and brain size, and increased risk of deformities of the genital and urinary organs. After birth, "crib death," or sudden unexplained death, may be more common in babies exposed to cocaine in utero. Children whose mothers used cocaine also have a high rate of behavioral difficulties, including hypersensitivity, irritability, and difficulty forming relationships. These children tend to do poorly in school and often have learning disabilities.

Research on pregnant cocaine users is difficult to perform, however, and many of the studies showing adverse effects on the fetus have methodological flaws that complicate the interpretation of their results. The major difficulty in studying pregnant women who use cocaine is the fact that a large percentage of these women also use other drugs or alcohol during their pregnancies. In addition, many of these women do not receive prenatal care and may be exposed to unhealthy or dangerous environments. We have known for many years that lack of prenatal care, by itself, leads to poor fetal outcome. Moreover, alcohol use has been documented to adversely affect the fetus. Therefore it is possible that not all of the negative effects reviewed above are caused by cocaine alone, or by cocaine at all. Although other factors besides cocaine use may be involved in causing fetal damage, there is clearly enough evidence to consider cocaine use during pregnancy extremely dangerous and, thus, to recommend very strongly against it. At the very least, we know that cocaine use during pregnancy is associated with a bad fetal outcome, even if it is unclear whether this is due to associated maternal malnutrition, polydrug use, and poor prenatal care or to a direct toxic effect of cocaine on the developing fetus.

Medical Complications Due to Drug Paraphernalia

Many of the medical difficulties that cocaine users experience are not caused by cocaine itself. Rather, they occur as a result of other factors that are as much a part of illicit cocaine use as the drug itself: drug paraphernalia and adulterants. The most hazardous of all drug paraphernalia is the unsterile needle. A needle is sterile if it is used only once after direct removal from a sterile package. Although this is the only method used in clinical medicine, sterile technique is far less common among intravenous drug users, who frequently use the same needle and syringe (commonly referred to as "a set of works") repeatedly because they are often expensive and sometimes difficult to obtain. An even more dangerous, but unfortunately common, method of needle use is that of sharing needles with other drug users. This practice can lead to a variety of very serious illnesses, including hepatitis and acquired immunodeficiency syndrome (AIDS).

Skin Infections

Perhaps the most common medical problem seen in intravenous cocaine users is infection of the skin and the tissues underneath the skin near injection sites. This occurs because an unsterile needle introduces bacteria beneath the outer layer of the skin, which normally acts as the body's first line of defense against infection. The introduction of bacteria into deeper layers of the skin may serve as a focus for infection. The most common manifestations of a skin infection include redness, swelling, heat, pain, and tenderness in the infected area. Spread of the infection may be detected by red streaks under the skin, signifying that the infection has spread to the lymphatic channels. If the infection is accompanied by fever, rapid heartbeat, and chills, then it may have spread into the bloodstream. This is an extremely serious sign, requiring immediate treatment, because it is potentially fatal if untreated. Although skin infections may seem rather benign, they deserve prompt medical attention because of their ability to spread rather quickly and cause serious damage both locally (e.g., infection of the tendon, joint, or bone) and in the rest of the body. Treatment for skin infections may consist of rest, moist heat, antibiotics, surgical drainage, or a combination of these treatments.

Endocarditis

Endocarditis, an infection of the heart valve, is one of the most serious infections that can develop in intravenous cocaine users. The disease develops when bacteria enter the bloodstream via unsterile needles and are deposited on a heart valve, where they may begin to multiply. These bacteria may then travel from the heart to other areas of the body, where they can cause great harm. For example, a shower of bacteria that lands in the lungs may cause a septic clot in the lung (pulmonary embolus), while a similar event in the brain may cause a stroke and a brain abscess. When endocarditis occurs in an intravenous drug user, the disease usually occurs acutely and progresses rapidly. High fever and chills are common. Abscesses may occur in the lungs, brain, or kidneys. When untreated, endocarditis is usually fatal. Some intravenous drug users, particularly heroin addicts, may misinterpret the fever and chills of endocarditis, believing that they are experiencing drug withdrawal. Many intravenous drug users ignore such manifestations of physical illness because of a general pattern of self-neglect and because of suspiciousness of physicians and hospitals. However, with appropriate treatment, which usually consists of at least four weeks of intravenous antibiotics, recovery may occur. The involved valve or valves may nevertheless sustain damage, perhaps necessitating surgical valve replacement at some future date.

Hepatitis

Hepatitis, or inflammation of the liver, is another very common disorder in cocaine users, particularly intravenous users. A New York study estimated that approximately two-thirds of intravenous drug users develop hepatitis at some point in their drug-abusing careers; two-thirds of this subpopulation contracts the disease within the first two years of injecting drugs. Thus the chance of an intravenous cocaine user developing hepatitis is approximately 50% within the first two years of drug use. Whereas hepatitis can be caused by a variety of agents—including alcohol, certain general anesthetics, and toxic chemicals—the most common form in cocaine users is caused by a virus that is transmitted from the blood of one user to that of another. Thus, hepatitis in cocaine users usually occurs as a result of sharing paraphernalia with other individuals who are already infected. Although the most common vehicle for the transmission of hepatitis in this population is a needle, there have been reports of hepatitis in exclusively intranasal cocaine users, perhaps caused by sharing straws, dollar bills, or "tooters" (thin glass or metal cylinders used for snorting cocaine) with other users. Because nosebleeds are commonly seen in active intranasal cocaine users, blood can easily be transmitted from one cocaine snorter to another; it takes less than a drop of contaminated blood to infect an other person with hepatitis.

The most serious (and occasionally fatal) form of hepatitis in drug users is hepatitis B, formerly termed *serum hepatitis*. One reason for the name change is the fact that hepatitis B can be transmitted via other means besides blood, such as through intimate sexual contact. However, infections in intravenous cocaine users are probably blood-borne in most cases. The disease is transmitted as follows: John, already infected with the hepatitis B virus, injects cocaine. Upon inserting the needle into his vein, the virus in his bloodstream contaminates the needle. This needle is then shared with Susan, who then injects the virus into her bloodstream along with her cocaine. After an incubation period ranging from one to six months (average is two to three months), the disease may strike.

Early symptoms of hepatitis vary widely and may include nausea, vomiting, headache, sore throat, cough, decreased appetite, fatigue, or joint pains. Patients with hepatitis often complain of an altered sense of taste or smell and may experience a darkening of their urine and/or a lightening of their stools, which may appear clay colored. An enlargement of the liver may occur during hepatitis; the liver, which is located under the right side of the rib cage, may become quite tender, especially during deep breathing. Jaundice, a yellow coloration of the skin or the whites of the eyes, may occur. Although this is considered by many drug users to be the hallmark of hepatitis, a significant number of patients with hepatitis never become jaundiced. Indeed, some people infected with the virus remain totally asymptomatic. Many intravenous users attempt to "protect" themselves against hepatitis by refusing to share a needle with a jaundiced drug user. Unfortunately, however, this rule of thumb is not an effective means of preventing hepatitis, both because of the long incubation period of hepatitis B (during which time the patient may be asymptomatic but still highly infectious) and because jaundice is not uniformly seen in patients who have hepatitis.

Recovery from hepatitis B generally occurs within 2 to 12 weeks, although fatigue may occur for even longer. Although the death rate from hepatitis B is estimated at less than 1%, chronic hepatitis may develop in up to 10% of all cases. Chronic hepatitis may progress to cirrhosis, a scarring of the liver that is sometimes fatal.

Hepatitis C is another form of viral hepatitis that can be transmitted like hepatitis B. Although it does not generally appear to have as serious a clinical course as hepatitis B, it is quite common in drug-dependent patients. Indeed, a recent study from Johns Hopkins University revealed that 86% of the intravenous drug users tested were positive for a history of hepatitis C—twice the prevalance rate of hepatitis B in the same population. Hepatitis A, which is transmitted through fecal material, is not necessarily more common in drug users than in other individuals.

Once an individual has developed hepatitis B, he or she generally develops antibodies to fight off the virus. The antibody may then provide protection against reinfection with the hepatitis B virus. Unfortunately, protection against hepatitis B does not provide immunity from future infection with hepatitis C. Many intravenous drug users are under the mistaken impression that after having hepatitis, they are henceforth immune to the disease. This is not true. Moreover, about 1% of individuals with hepatitis B do not develop antibodies and remain chronic carriers of the virus (i.e., they remain chronically infectious). This chronic carrier state may or may not be associated with chronic hepatitis.

There is no specific treatment for acute viral hepatitis. For individuals who have recently been exposed to the hepatitis B virus, an injection of hepatitis B immune globulin (HBIG) may be recommended to decrease the likelihood and seriousness of the disease. Otherwise, the best advice is to eat and sleep well and to avoid contact with alcohol (a liver toxin) and needles. Despite the lack of specific treatments for hepatitis B, a hepatitis B vaccine offers excellent protection against the disease.

AIDS

In 1981, the medical community first filed reports of a heretofore unreported syndrome now known as *AIDS*. At that time, previously healthy homosexual men were developing an extremely rare tumor known as Kaposi's sarcoma, as well as a form of pneumonia (*Pneumocystis carinii*) that is generally seen only in patients with severely compromised immune systems. Since the early 1980s, it is estimated that more than one million individuals in the United States have been infected with the virus that causes AIDS, known as the *human immunodeficiency virus (HIV)*. Currently, AIDS is considered a fatal disease, although with newly developed treatments, individuals are living increasingly longer after infection.

AIDS is caused by infection with HIV. Like the hepatitis B and C viruses, HIV can be transmitted through needle sharing or blood-to-blood contact. The virus is also present in semen, cervical and vaginal secretions, and saliva, which means that sexual contact is another major way the virus is transmitted. Activities that place an individual at high risk of contracting HIV from an infected person include anal or vaginal intercourse without a condom, unprotected oral sex (fellatio or cunnilingus), blood contact of any kind, and sharing needles or sex instruments. Using a condom dramatically decreases the risk of contracting HIV through intercourse.

Although AIDS was initially seen most often in homosexual men, the incidence of AIDS infection in intravenous drug users has been steadily increasing. Currently, approximately 25% to 30% of all people with AIDS are intravenous drug users. HIV infection is spreading so quickly in this population that some cities estimate that almost half of their intravenous drug users are now infected. Furthermore, recent studies have shown that intravenous users of cocaine may be at especially high risk. Dr. Richard Chaisson and co-workers found that 35% of daily intravenous cocaine users in San Francisco were infected with HIV—a higher prevalence rate than seen in intravenous users of other drugs, such as heroin. The researchers hypothesized that this was due to the fact that cocaine users may inject their drug more frequently (up to 10 times a day or more) than do users of other drugs, thus increasing the number of times that they could be exposed to HIV. Other aspects of the life-style of individuals addicted to cocaine, such as the use of drugs in shooting galleries and the exchange of cocaine for sex, may also increase the spread of HIV.

HIV testing.   Blood testing for antibodies to HIV is the only available method of determining whether someone has been infected. After the virus is introduced into the body, it takes 6 to 12 weeks for antibodies to develop in most people. These antibodies can then be detected by a blood test. In some people, however, antibodies do not develop for six months after infection. In these cases, an HIV test would be negative even though an individual had contracted the virus and could transmit it to others. A new method known as *polymerase chain reaction (PCR) testing* tests for the presence of the virus itself, rather than the antibody. With this testing technique, one could determine much sooner after exposure whether an individual had indeed become infected with HIV. At the time of this writing, PCR testing was still experimental.

Symptoms of HIV infection.   As far as we know, most people who contract HIV eventually develop AIDS, although it may take up to 10 years or more for symptoms of AIDS to appear. Initial infection with HIV may result in a flu-like syndrome consisting of body aches, fever, and gastrointestinal symptoms that may last two to three weeks. After this syndrome has resolved, an individual may be asymptomatic for months to years before developing signs of AIDS. Over time, the virus damages the immune system by invading and destroying blood cells. White blood cells known as *T4 lymphocytes* are particularly damaged by the virus, rendering the body unable to fight off other infections. As a person's immune system becomes weaker, he or she may begin to get infections that do not typically occur in healthy people; this generally means that an individual has developed AIDS.

Symptoms of AIDS. An individual with AIDS is at risk of getting a wide range of infections, many of which can be lethal. A form of pneumonia known as *Pneumocystis carinii* is particularly common. In addition, opportunistic infections of the brain (meningitis or encephalitis), liver (hepatitis), mouth (oropharyngitis), or gastrointestinal tract can occur. Certain forms of cancer (e.g., Kaposi's sarcoma and lymphoma) are also frequent in AIDS. Ultimately, death occurs in individuals with AIDS, usually from overwhelming infection.

Treatment of AIDS. There is currently no cure for AIDS. Infections can be treated with antibiotics, and precautions can be taken to prevent further infections. Two drugs, zidovudine (AZT) and dideoxyinosine (DDI), have been clearly shown to slow down the progression of AIDS. Unfortunately, these medications do not prevent AIDS from developing, nor do they prevent AIDS from being ultimately fatal. There are many other experimental drugs now being tested, however, that may prove more effective in treating AIDS in the future.

Medical Complications Due to Adulterants ("Cuts")

Although cocaine itself can produce a wide variety of medical and psychological problems in users, street "cocaine" presents additional hazards. Because illicitly purchased cocaine may be as little as 10% pure, up to 90% of the product being snorted, smoked, or injected is present only because it either looks, tastes, or feels like cocaine. These adulterants (cuts) can cause much of the toxicity that cocaine users experience.

One of the problems that intravenous drug users frequently encounter is lung damage due to the frequent injection of adulterants such as talc or starch. Researchers have hypothesized that the injection of these adulterants obstructs small blood vessels in the lungs, causing an inflammatory reaction (granulomatous lung disease). This is typically a persistent, smoldering area of inflammation that may last for months or longer, even after the cessation of drug use. It has been estimated that 25% to 70% of intravenous drug users have such abnormalities in their lungs. These abnormalities can occur even in the absence of symptoms, such as shortness of breath or cough, that one would ordinarily expect in patients with lung disease.

Medical Complications Due to Life-Style and Psychiatric Symptoms in Cocaine Users

Polysubstance Use

Most users of cocaine also use other illicit drugs or alcohol. Some estimates have placed the number of individuals addicted to cocaine who use other substances as high as 90%. Alcohol is commonly used by cocaine users to "smooth out" their cocaine "high" or to decrease undesirable effects of cocaine, such as irritability or anxiety. Recent data have revealed that the combination of cocaine and alcohol may be particularly hazardous. A University of Miami research group, led by Dr. William Hearn, have discovered that when an individual uses alcohol along with cocaine, the breakdown of cocaine in the body is altered, producing a new compound called *cocaethylene*. Early evidence from animal research suggests that cocaethylene may be more toxic (particularly to the heart) than cocaine alone. Moreover, cocathylene remains in the body approximately three times as long as cocaine. Thus combining cocaine with alcohol may lead to a higher rate of serious (sometimes fatal) medical complications.

In addition to alcohol, other drugs such as diazepam (Valium), barbiturates, alprazolam (Xanax), marijuana, or heroin may be used along with cocaine, often for similar reasons. Unfortunately, the combined effects of these drugs is often more dangerous than the effects of any one drug alone. The risks of medical complications, suicide, homicide, and accidents are greatly increased with polydrug use. In addition, polysubstance use has become common in pregnant cocaine users as discussed earlier.

Suicide

Another group of health hazards resulting from long-term cocaine use occurs because of the psychiatric effects of cocaine and the lifestyle that frequently accompanies its use. As we have discussed, cocaine can cause roller coaster–like swings between euphoria and depression. As the frequency and intensity of cocaine use increase, the severity of the depression can increase proportionately. Some cocaine users become suicidal as a result of the neurochemical depression caused by the drug and because of the sense of hopelessness that they may experience after repeated unsuccessful attempts to stop their drug use. Thus the risk of suicide represents another potential medical danger for cocaine users.

Accidents

In addition to the accidental deaths that can occur as the result of an unintentional overdose, automobile accidents are much more likely to occur among long-term cocaine users. Cocaine users often feel a sense of invincibility that may encourage them to drive faster and more recklessly than they ordinarily would. This can occur even in occasional users and is not merely the result of long-term cocaine use. A study of motor vehicle fatalities in New York City conducted by Dr. Peter Marzuk and co-workers found that 18% of all people killed in car accidents had cocaine in their bodies at autopsy. Both alcohol and cocaine were found in 10% of these cases, meaning 8% had used cocaine alone. (Another 38% had just alcohol in their bodies.) This suggests that cocaine use, by itself, does impair one's ability to drive safely. When combined with alcohol or other drugs like Valium, which have been clearly shown to impair driving ability, cocaine users are at extremely high risk of having accidents.

Homicide

A final cause of death in cocaine users is murder. Homicide may occur for several reasons. First, cocaine is illegal. Thus to obtain it, users must deal with criminals. Although some cocaine users initially buy their drugs from friends in small quantities, the dangerousness of their contacts often increases as their drug habit escalates. Many prospective cocaine buyers frequently enter into dangerous situations while carrying large sums of money, thus presenting inviting targets for robbery, mugging, or homicide. In addition, because large doses of cocaine often produce paranoia, heavy users may attempt to defend themselves against real or imagined enemies by obtaining weapons. Such was the case with John, a 27-year-old man who had been using cocaine for two years:

> After a while, I was convinced that there were people trying to break into my house. I didn't know who they were, but I was sure that people were after me. There was probably some reality to it too, since I really was scared that the police would come in and bust me. The only way that I felt that I could protect myself was by getting a knife. So I started sleeping with a butcher knife next to me. That didn't work for long, though, because I still felt insecure. So I felt that I had to get a gun. Every night, I went to bed with a gun on one side of me and a butcher knife on the other side. I was just waiting for someone to come in the house so that I could blow his brains out. God knows what I was going to do with the knife. I swear, I was a maniac. It wouldn't have mattered who had come to the door. If someone had come to my door at the wrong time to borrow a cup of sugar, I can tell you with 100% certainty, he would have been dead.

Clearly, a person such as John, whose story is not unusual, is also a target for other paranoid cocaine users with whom he or she is dealing. This combination of extremely poor judgment, paranoia, intermittent crippling depression, and a stockpiling of lethal weapons may lead to violent deaths in an unfortunate number of long-term cocaine users.

Chapter 4

Cocaine and the Brain

The widespread popularity of cocaine reflects the drug's powerful effects on the brain and, consequently, on behavior. However, although cocaine is highly valued for its ability to produce euphoria, enhance alertness, and alleviate fatigue, many users think very little about the drug's long-term effects on mood. In this chapter we describe both the short- and long-term effects of cocaine on brain function. This information is based on research carried out on both animal and human subjects, as well as on the accumulated experience of over 1,500 years of cocaine consumption.

Basic Elements of Brain Function: The Nerve Cell

Understanding the effects of cocaine (or any drug) on brain function first requires some knowledge about how the brain works. The brain consists of a collection of nerve cells called *neurons,* which are unique among all cells of the body in that they are specially adapted to receive and dispatch electrical impulses. Neurons are able to accomplish this because of their unique anatomical and physiological characteristics.

As shown in Figure 1, the typical nerve cell has a system of branches, called *dendrites,* whose specialized surfaces are equipped to receive incoming electrical signals from other neurons. These signals, in turn, are conveyed to the main body of the nerve cell, where new electrical impulses are generated. Outgoing impulses travel down a part of the cell called the *axon,* whose endings, called *terminal boutons* (or *synaptic buttons*), are specialized for the transmission of these impulses to other neurons. Axons may be long or short, and may either end locally or travel to other regions of the central nervous system and beyond. For example, neurons whose cell bodies are up in the cerebral cortex or brain stem may extend their long axons down into the spinal cord. These axons join there with other nerve cells, whose axons in turn travel out of the spinal cord to connect with muscles and body organs.

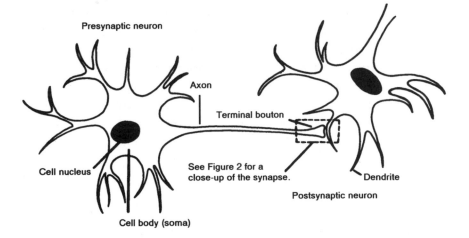

Figure 1. Synaptic connection between two neurons. Neurotransmitter precursors are commonly synthesized in the cell body of the presynaptic neuron and transported down the axon to the terminal bouton where they are produced and stored in vesicles. An action potential traveling down the axon causes release of the neurotransmitter into the narrow space between the two neurons, the synaptic cleft. Many axons terminate adjacent to dendrites of the postsynaptic neuron, as shown here. This is know as an *axondendritic synapse.* Some axons terminate on the postsynaptic cell body (*axosomatic synapses*), and others terminate on other axons (*axoaxonic synapses*). *Source.* Reprinted from Martin MB, Owen CM, Morihisa JM: "An Overview of Neurotransmitters and Neuroreceptors," in *The American Psychiatric Press Textbook of Neuropsychiatry.* Edited by Hales RE, Yudofsky SC. Washington, DC, American Psychiatric Press, 1987, p. 57. Used with permission.

The area of interface between two nerve cells is called a *synapse*. In the following section, we briefly describe the events that occur at this junction, because an understanding of the synapse is crucial to understanding the effects of cocaine on mood and behavior.

Events at the Nerve Cell Junction (Synapse)

The synapse plays a critical role in the central nervous system because it is here that information is conveyed from one nerve cell to another. In those few areas of the brain in which nerve cells are extremely close together, synapses are *electrotonic,* which means that electrical impulses are transmitted directly from neuron to neuron, much like an electrical current traveling down a connected wire. In the vast majority of synapses, however, chemical substances called *neurotransmitters* transport the electrical messages across the gaps that separate nerve cells.

A number of chemical compounds have been identified as neurotransmitters in the central nervous system. From the standpoint of our discussion of cocaine, the most important of these are *dopamine, norepinephrine, and serotonin.* Like other transmitters, these compounds are stored in tiny sacs called *vesicles,* which are clustered in the terminal bouton of the nerve cell (see Figure 2). In response to electrical changes on the surface of the nerve cell, these neurotransmitters are released into the synaptic space (cleft) between neurons. The neuron that releases a neurotransmitter is designated as the *presynaptic* neuron. The neuron that receives these transmitter molecules is the *postsynaptic* neuron. Almost every nerve cell functions as both a pre- and postsynaptic neuron, depending on its relationship to its neighboring nerve cells.

Transmission of an electrical impulse across the synapse occurs as follows: When the nerve impulse traveling down the axon reaches the synaptic button, the vesicles migrate to the cell wall and spill their neurotransmitters into the synaptic space. These neurotransmitters are then free to attach to specialized receptors on the surface of the target (postsynaptic) cell. The attachment of neurotransmitters to these receptors on the target cell upsets the electrical balance in the latter by allowing certain electrically charged ions like sodium, potassium, chloride, and calcium to cross the target cell membrane. This membrane is a semipermeable barrier that separates the inside of the nerve cell from the surrounding "extracellular" fluid. The electrical shift in the postsynaptic nerve cell may cause the cell to "fire," thus resulting in transmission of the electri-

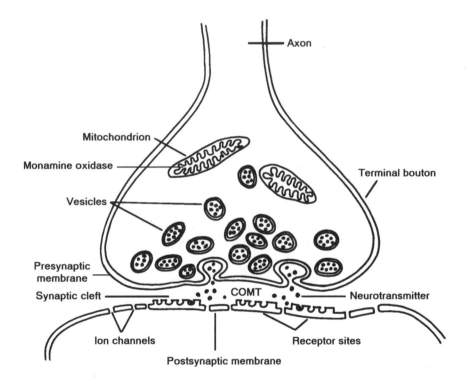

Figure 2. Close-up of a synapse. Molecules of neurotransmitter are enclosed in vesicles in the terminal bouton of the axon. Two vesicles are shown fused to the presynaptic membrane, releasing neurotransmitters into the synaptic cleft. The neurotransmitter initiates activity in the postsynaptic neuron by biding to receptor sites in the postsynaptic membrane. COMT = catechol-O-methyltransferase. *Source.* Reprinted from Martin MB, Owen CM, Morihisa JM: "An Overview of Neurotransmitters and Neuroreceptors," in *The American Psychiatric Press Textbook of Neuropsychiatry.* Edited by Hales RE, Yudofsky SC. Washington, DC, American Psychiatric Press, 1987, p. 58. Used with permission.

cal impulse down its own axon. This entire process is constantly occurring in neurons located in all areas of the brain.

The functional result of neurotransmitter release depends on the effect each neurotransmitter has on its particular postsynaptic neuron. Some neurotransmitters are *excitatory,* in that they facilitate transmission of an electrical impulse as described above. Others are *inhibitory* in that their effect on postsynaptic nerve cells makes neuronal firing less likely. Because every nerve cell may receive either excitatory or inhibitory input from surrounding neurons, firing of a particular cell occurs only when the net accumulation of all of that cell's input reaches its threshold level.

The chemical reactions at the postsynaptic receptor are followed by release of the neurotransmitter compounds back into the synaptic space. There, one of two processes serves to end the reaction. The transmitters may be metabolized (broken down) by chemicals called *enzymes*—the most important of which is called *catechol-O-methyltransferase (COMT)*. Alternatively, the transmitters are returned to the presynaptic neuron, a process called *reuptake*. There the transmitters are broken down by enzymes inside the cell, particularly *monoamine oxidase (MAO)* (see Figure 2).

Effects of Cocaine on Neurotransmitters

Neurotransmitters are broken down into a variety of metabolic end products that can be measured in urine, blood, and cerebrospinal fluid. The ability to measure these metabolic end products can sometimes help researchers investigate the effects of drugs like cocaine on the production, release, and breakdown of various neurotransmitters.

Another way of measuring the direct effects of cocaine and other drugs on the brain is through the use of new brain imaging techniques such as single photon emission computed tomography (SPECT), positron-emission tomography (PET), and topographic brain mapping (e.g., brain electrical activity mapping [BEAM]). These techniques can assess brain functioning by using a computer to generate color-coded maps of brain activity. PET scanning, for example, has allowed scientists to "visualize" the receptors for dopamine in the brains of cocaine-addicted patients. PET scanning can also be used to measure changes in glucose metabolism and cerebral blood flow during cocaine use, whereas topographic brain mapping monitors rapid changes in the neuronal activity described in the previous section. Studies using these imaging techniques have shown that cocaine users typically have one or more areas of abnormal metabolism, cerebral blood flow, or brain functioning compared with subjects who do not use drugs.

Although the implications of such findings are still not well understood, there has been progress in understanding the mechanism of cocaine's effects. Experimental evidence to date suggests that cocaine, as well as other central nervous system stimulants such as amphetamine, affects levels of dopamine, norepinephrine, and serotonin. It appears that cocaine inhibits the reuptake of these neurotransmitters back into the presynaptic neuron after they have been released into the synapse. Prevention of reuptake effectively increases the availability of these neurotransmitters in the synapse. In addition, cocaine may directly stimulate the release of dopamine and norepinephrine into the synapse. This increased availability of neurotransmitters is thought to be essential to the acute behavioral and psychological effects of cocaine. Another mechanism of action of cocaine is related to its effect on the receptors for neurotransmitters. With chronic use, the sensitivity of dopamine receptors is altered. These receptor changes may be involved in the development of *tolerance* and *withdrawal,* phenomena that are discussed later in this chapter.

Additional evidence points to the particular importance of dopamine in cocaine abuse and dependence. A recent study by Dr. Mary Ritz and co-workers, for example, found that inhibition of dopamine reuptake was associated with increased cocaine self-administration in monkeys. This effect was not seen with inhibition of norepinephrine or serotonin reuptake. Because the interrelationships of neurotransmitters are complex, however, we certainly have more to learn about the roles of norepinephrine, serotonin, and perhaps other brain chemicals in cocaine dependence. For the purposes of this chapter, we will focus on the effects of cocaine on dopamine and, to some extent, on norepinephrine, which are thought to be important in the regulation of behavior, mood, level of consciousness, motor function, and hormonal output.

Effects of Cocaine on Brain Function and Behavior

Effects on Consciousness and Arousal

In both animals and humans, cocaine causes increased alertness and enhanced mental acuity when first administered, accompanied by marked changes in brain electrical activity. One area of the brain that is particularly affected by cocaine is the reticular formation, a nerve network running through portions of the brain stem that is thought to be involved in the regulation of consciousness, attention, and arousal.

The increased arousal and diminished need for sleep observed after cocaine use appears to be associated with the effects of the drug on certain central nervous system neurons that are thought to have an activating effect on human behavior. As described above, cocaine blocks the return (reuptake) of neurotransmitters from the synaptic space back into the presynaptic neuron (thus interfering with their metabolic breakdown); the drug may also increase the release of dopamine and norepinephrine into the synapse. These actions increase the availability of norepinephrine and dopamine in the synapse and therefore increase nerve cell firing in areas of the brain that control wakefulness and arousal.

Cocaine and the Perception of Pleasure

Dopamine is a neurotransmitter that has been linked to pleasure, so it is not surprising that it may also be involved in the repeated use of cocaine. In other words, cocaine, apparently through its effect on dopamine, functions as a powerful "reinforcer." The major site of action of cocaine on the dopamine system is in an area of the brain called the *nucleus accumbens.* This is in contrast with opiates, also potent reinforcers, which probably act in an area called the *ventral tegmentum,* another part of the brain that contains dopamine-producing neurons. The primary reinforcing effects of both cocaine and opiates appear to be independent of their ability to induce physical dependence. Thus the need in some users to repeat the drug experience is caused more by the pursuit of euphoria than by a desire to ameliorate symptoms of drug withdrawal.

The reinforcing effect of cocaine has been demonstrated clearly in laboratory animals such as rats and monkeys. Once they have become acquainted with its euphoria-inducing effects, these animals will perform "work" such as repetitively pressing a lever to receive injections of cocaine. In fact, animals will choose cocaine over food and water, and they will continue to seek cocaine even if they are "punished" for using it. One study has even shown that if the availability of cocaine is unlimited, monkeys will use cocaine excessively to the point of severe toxicity and death. This finding is consistent with the drug's appeal in humans and the tendency of users to want to repeat the drug experience. Some researchers have speculated that this phenomenon is due to the effects of cocaine on certain "reward" areas of the brain, which are responsible for the perception of pleasure.

Although the brain mechanisms underlying cocaine's reinforcing properties are complex, a number of studies have shown that its effect on dopamine levels is essential. Drugs that act like dopamine, known as *dopamine agonists,* tend to be reinforcers themselves. In other words, animals will self-administer dopamine agonists just as they will self-administer cocaine. The role of dopamine has been further verified in laboratory rats by administering drugs that destroy either norepinephrine-secreting or dopamine-secreting neurons and then allowing the animals to self-administer intravenous cocaine. In a 1977 study, destruction of those nerve pathways that use norepinephrine as a neurotransmitter failed to interfere with the reinforcing effects of cocaine. In other words, these animals continued to work for cocaine injections despite the lack of norepinephrine-mediated activity in their brains. In contrast, destruction of those neurons that use dopamine as a neurotransmitter resulted in a significant and long-lasting decrease in cocaine self-administration behavior. This early study has been replicated by more recent research. In 1988, Drs. Steven Dworkin and James Smith were able to show that destruction of dopamine-producing neurons in the nucleus accumbens decreased cocaine's reinforcing effects. Recent research has suggested that these dopamine-mediated reinforcing effects are not unique to cocaine use, but may affect opiate use as well. This area of study continues to be explored.

In summary, it appears that dopamine-containing neurons play an important role in mediating the positive reinforcing properties of cocaine. There is evidence that opiate drugs also exert their reinforcing effects by activating dopamine-containing neurons in the brain, although opiates and cocaine apparently act at different locations in the brain and perhaps through different mechanisms.

Stereotyped Behavior

Since the beginning of this century, cocaine users have been noted to sometimes exhibit compulsive stereotyped behaviors. Some long-term users, for instance, may spend hours taking apart radios or television sets and putting them back together. Other similarly meaningless compulsive behaviors, particularly those requiring attention to detail, may also be observed in these individuals. A recent report has also shown that individuals with obsessive-compulsive disorder may experience a worsening of their compulsive behaviors when they use cocaine.

The cause of these stereotyped behaviors is thought to be related to alterations in neurotransmitters, especially dopamine. Prior administration of alpha-methylparatyrosine (AMPT), a drug that inhibits the production of norepinephrine and dopamine, will prevent the development of stereotyped behavior in animals. This suggests that these neurotransmitters are involved in producing this compulsive behavior.

Sensitization and Kindling

In animals, repeated dosing of cocaine increases hyperactivity, stereotyped behaviors, and sometimes causes seizures. This phenomenon is known as *sensitization*. This is in contrast to *tolerance,* which refers to a decrease in drug effects with repeated dosing. Sensitization is thought to occur as a result of the effects of cocaine on dopamine-containing neurons in parts of the brain that control motor activity. Sensitization can only occur if cocaine is administered intermittently, and not constantly, for reasons that are not well understood.

Another important factor in sensitization is environmental conditioning. For example, if a drug is given in the presence of other "nondrug" cues or stimuli, then presenting these conditioned stimuli alone can eventually evoke some of the responses observed after administration of the drug alone. Dr. Robert Post and colleagues at the National Institute of Mental Health showed that rats can be conditioned by the environment of cocaine administration. One group of rats was given cocaine in a "test" cage and another group given the drug in their "home" cage. Later, all the rats were placed in the test cage and given additional cocaine. The rats who had previously received cocaine in the test cage showed more hyperactive behavior than the other group: these rats were manifesting greater sensitization to the drug, because they were now receiving it in a location previously associated with cocaine administration. It appears that dopamine is essential to the acquisition of these conditioned behaviors. The effects of conditioned stimuli (i.e., the environmental cues that help to produce the response previously associated only with drug use) can be diminished if dopamine-blocking drugs, such as neuroleptics, are given to animals in similar test conditions.

The concept of sensitization is useful in understanding why long-time cocaine users may become increasingly hyperactive or may develop stereotyped, compulsive behaviors. Seizures can also occur with chronic cocaine use, probably as a result of kindling. *Kindling* is the process by which repeated electrical stimulation of the brain eventually leads to the development of seizures. As with sensitization, these stimuli must be given intermittently and not continuously. Each stimulus by itself is not large enough to produce a seizure. Cocaine is thought to produce "pharmacological kindling," leading to seizures in some chronic users.

The mechanism of cocaine-induced kindling has been studied in laboratory animals. Neurons repeatedly exposed to cocaine become sensitized to the effects of the drug and thus fire more readily with each succeeding drug exposure. During long-term use, these neurons fire even in response to relatively low doses of the drug. At the same time, abnormal electrical activity can be detected in the *limbic system,* an area of the brain known to regulate emotions. This abnormal brain activity can spread outside the emotional centers of the brain to cause generalized (grand mal) seizures.

In rhesus monkeys, for example, long-term administration of cocaine (e.g., over a six-month period) results in a progressive increase in pathological behavior, even in animals maintained on a fixed dose of the drug. Initially, the animals display the typical hyperactivity and stereotyped behavior observed in other species. After two months of cocaine use, however, they begin to demonstrate slowed movements, bizarre postures, staring, and a diminished ability to track objects in space. Some of these animals develop signs that suggest abnormalities in those nerve pathways that regulate voluntary and involuntary movement. Many also demonstrate an increased susceptibility to seizures, which is due to the tendency of cocaine to increase the electrical excitability of the brain. Indeed, there is evidence that before the onset of seizures in these animals, well-defined abnormalities of brain electrical activity may be observed, especially in the limbic system. These abnormal electrical discharges in the limbic system may also account for the behavioral changes observed during long-term, high-dose cocaine use in both animals and humans. Prior administration of a drug like carbamazepine (Tegretol), which lowers the level of electrical activity in the limbic system, will prevent the development of seizures and other types of abnormal behavior in these animals.

The phenomenon of kindling has also been hypothesized to be involved in some of the adverse psychiatric effects of long-term cocaine use. For example, kindling may partially explain the development of cocaine psychosis that can occur with repeated cocaine use.

Cocaine psychosis is discussed more fully at the end of this chapter. Some researchers have also suggested that kindling may also explain why some cocaine users develop panic attacks.

In summary, long-term cocaine use appears to generate a form of pharmacological kindling that may account for the increased sensitivity of long-term users to the acute effects of the drug. Indeed, in some cases, the brain response to cocaine may be permanently altered. This would explain why, even after a long period of abstinence, individuals who had previously developed psychological difficulties as the result of long-term cocaine use may rapidly return to their cocaine-induced state even if exposed to extremely low doses of the drug.

Tolerance

Although repeated cocaine use can lead to sensitization to the development of motor hyperactivity and stereotyped behaviors, *tolerance* may develop to other effects of cocaine. As mentioned earlier, tolerance occurs when repeated drug use leads to a decrease in the drug's effects. A recent study by Dr. John Ambre and co-workers has shown that tolerance develops to the euphoric and cardiovascular effects of the drug. These researchers gave a group of regular cocaine users continuous infusions of cocaine, during which they measured heart rate and subjective reports of euphoria. They found that complete tolerance developed to the subjective effects. Specifically, subjects given the same dose of cocaine no longer experienced euphoria over time. Tolerance to the cardiovascular effects over time was only partial; the subjects' heart rates decreased, but did not return to normal. The mechanism of tolerance is hypothesized to be caused by receptor changes as a result of continuous drug use.

These findings have significance in understanding why cocaine users on a "run" may eventually no longer feel euphoric with repeated doses. If the users respond by increasing their dose in an attempt to overcome the tolerance to euphoria, they may be placing themselves at great risk for a toxic reaction.

Behavioral Effects of Long-Term Cocaine Use

Cocaine and Depression

Although cocaine initially produces euphoria, many otherwise nondepressed users experience depression and anxiety after repeated high-dose use. These effects have also been noted in some individuals during long-term use of other central nervous system stimulants like amphetamine or methylphenidate (Ritalin). Some long-term cocaine users simultaneously take central nervous system depressants (barbiturates, benzodiazepines, or alcohol) or even opioids in an attempt to reduce their dysphoria and anxiety.

As early as 1974, there was evidence that cocaine does not make everyone euphoric. Dr. Robert Post and his colleagues speculated that cocaine may exert antidepressant activity; they thus explored the effects of cocaine in clinically depressed individuals. Although some patients did experience a brief period of euphoria following intravenous cocaine use, others became more depressed. With continued use, particularly at high doses, the majority of patients became quite tearful, anxious, and distraught.

Since Dr. Post's early study, more evidence has accumulated that demonstrates a link between cocaine use and depression. Dr. Bruce Rounsaville and his co-workers at Yale University found that more than 50% of the cocaine-dependent patients they studied had been significantly depressed at some point in their lives. Furthermore, about two-thirds of these depressed individuals reported that their depression began after they started to use cocaine. Studies by our research group at McLean Hospital in Belmont, Massachusetts, have also revealed a high prevalence rate of mood disorders in this population. Thus it appears that the use of cocaine is associated with the development of depression. We do not know, however, how much of this depression is caused by the long-term effects of cocaine on the brain, how much is due to the social disruption and losses frequently associated with cocaine use, and how much is due to a preexisting condition. Moreover, the cessation of cocaine use is also associated with depressive symptoms that may be confused with depression caused by other factors.

Depression ("crashing") following cessation of cocaine use is a fairly common phenomenon in both novice and experienced users. Although this may occur even after only a short bout with low doses of the drug, it is most common after stopping long-term, high-dose cocaine use. In 1986, Drs. Frank Gawin and Herbert Kleber published the first systematic study describing the *cocaine abstinence syndrome*. They found that during the first one to three days of abstinence, users typically experience depression, irritability, anxiety, confusion, insomnia, and a gradually diminishing desire for more cocaine. This is followed by a one- to three-day period of depression, apathy, lethargy, increased appetite, and an enormous desire for sleep. Interestingly, this phase of the crash is often accompanied by an aversion to cocaine.

Following the initial crash, a phase that Gawin and Kleber called *cocaine withdrawal* begins. This phase is roughly analogous to withdrawal from other substances, such as alcohol, except that most symptoms are experienced as psychological rather than somatic. In the withdrawal phase, newly abstinent users typically spend one to five days in which they feel good, sleep normally, and experience little craving for cocaine because of their strong recognition of the drug's adverse effects. However, this period of calm may soon give way to another bout of depression, anxiety, irritability, lethargy, and severe boredom, frequently accompanied by a renewal of intense craving for cocaine. Over the next one to four days, bad memories about cocaine are gradually replaced by recollections of the drug's euphoric effects. Under these circumstances, if cocaine is available, relapse frequently occurs. This period of depression, lethargy, and disinterest can last, sometimes at subtle levels, for at least two months.

More recent research has challenged the idea that cocaine abstinence occurs in several phases. Dr. William Weddington and his colleagues at the National Institute on Drug Abuse, for instance, found that cocaine addicts experienced their greatest distress and drug craving right after admission to treatment and improved on these measures gradually but steadily during a four-week inpatient program. Therefore, although depression and drug craving are commonly seen in individuals who have recently stopped using cocaine, the etiology, severity, and time course of these symptoms are controversial.

Some researchers have posited that the biological mechanisms underlying the depression that frequently occurs during cocaine withdrawal are related to the effects of the drug on brain neurotransmitters. As described above, cocaine blocks the reuptake of dopamine into neurons, leading to increased availability of dopamine. Increased dopamine in areas of the brain associated with pleasure is thought to be associated with cocaine's reinforcing properties and its euphoric effects. With chronic use of cocaine, however, this dopamine response is altered and perhaps decreased. The etiology of altered dopamine dynamics is still unclear, but it may be related to changes in dopamine receptors or changes in other neurotransmitters that affect dopamine. If, in fact, dopamine release is decreased in areas of the brain that are associated with pleasure, this could explain why chronic cocaine users might feel depressed when not using cocaine. Clarifying the brain changes associated with chronic cocaine use and cocaine withdrawal remains a focus of ongoing research.

Finally, it is important to note that cocaine is not the only drug of abuse associated with depression. Depression commonly develops in users of alcohol and opioids, for example. It has been hypothesized that drugs other than cocaine may also affect dopamine-mediated "reward" pathways in the brain as a "final common pathway." Whether this means that there is a common etiology for the depression that frequently occurs in alcohol, opioid, and cocaine users has not been determined.

Cocaine Psychosis

As the dose and duration of cocaine use increase, the euphoria associated with the drug often disappears, and is replaced by depression, irritability, and, in some cases, psychosis. Epidemiological studies show that paranoia and other psychotic symptoms are most common in individuals who use cocaine daily; casual use does not typically lead to paranoid thinking. Smoking crack cocaine appears to be the route of use most commonly associated with paranoia, perhaps because the frequency of use is usually higher with crack use than with intranasal or intravenous use.

Cocaine psychosis is typically preceded by a transitional period that is characterized by increased suspiciousness, compulsive behavior, and dysphoric mood. Users also become increasingly irritable, fault finding, and eventually quite paranoid. Some psychotic individuals experience visual and/or auditory hallucinations, with persecutory "voices" commonly heard. They may also feel that they are being followed by the police or that others are plotting against them. Everyday events may be misinterpreted in a way that supports these paranoid beliefs. When coupled with irritability and hyperactivity, cocaine-induced paranoia may lead to violent behavior as a means of "self-defense" against imagined persecutors. Individuals with cocaine psychosis may also experience tactile hallucinations. Some users, for instance, develop the belief that they have parasites ("cocaine bugs") crawling under their skin. These individuals may pick constantly at their skin and produce open sores.

The development of paranoia during cocaine use appears to be common. Dr. Sally Satel and her colleagues at Yale University studied 50 cocaine-dependent patients and found that 68% had developed transient paranoia during binge cocaine use. Most of these individuals reported that their paranoia worsened with continued cocaine use; all but one reported that the paranoia dissipated when cocaine use ceased. Typical paranoid thoughts included the fear of attack by others and the suspicion that police or drug dealers were about to apprehend them. Many patients reported that they acted on their paranoid thoughts, for example, by hiding in a closet for fear of being caught by the police or by arming themselves with a weapon. Interestingly, not everyone who used large amounts of cocaine for long periods of time developed paranoid symptoms. These researchers suggested that some cocaine users may be predisposed to becoming paranoid, perhaps because of other drug use, family history, or other biological and social factors.

In searching for the underlying cause of cocaine psychosis, we are led again to the effects of the drug on brain neurotransmitters. In this regard, it is important to note that in patients with non–drug-induced psychosis, such as schizophrenia, there is evidence of increased activity of those central nervous system neurons that use dopamine as a neurotransmitter. High doses of cocaine and other central nervous system stimulants also appear to increase the firing rate of dopamine-containing neurons in the brain. During long-term cocaine use, for example, homovanillic acid, the major breakdown product of dopamine, is elevated in the cerebrospinal fluid of laboratory animals. This may be the result of cocaine-induced release of dopamine from presynaptic neurons or the drug's interference with the reuptake of this neurotransmitter into presynaptic neurons and its metabolic breakdown.

A recent study by Dr. Michael Sherer demonstrated a correlation between elevated dopamine levels and paranoia in cocaine users. He studied eight intravenous cocaine users by giving them continuous cocaine infusions over a period of four hours. After two hours, subjects became increasingly suspicious, and one developed hallucinations. In all but one individual, these paranoid symptoms resolved within hours after cocaine administration stopped; one subject was still suspicious the following day. Dr. Sherer showed that suspiciousness and paranoia were related to an increase in homovanillic acid, suggesting that paranoia in these subjects was related to increased levels of dopamine in the brain.

To summarize, long-term cocaine use appears to increase the activity of dopamine-containing neurons, and the development of stimulant-induced psychosis appears to be correlated with excessive levels of brain dopamine activity. Most researchers believe that this is also the underlying cause of the stereotyped behavior seen in both animals and humans after long-term cocaine use. Consistent with this hypothesis, the treatment of cocaine psychosis entails withdrawal of the drug and, in emergencies, the administration of psychoactive medications that block the effects of dopamine in postsynaptic neurons. Such drugs, called *neuroleptics,* are also effective in the treatment of schizophrenia and manic states, suggesting that increased brain dopamine may be an important factor in these conditions as well.

Cocaine and Cognitive Functioning

A recent study by Dr. Stephanie O'Malley of Yale University and her colleagues revealed a mild but definite impairment in cognitive functioning in a group of 20 heavy cocaine users. These impairments were revealed by a battery of neuropsychological tests that measure a wide variety of cognitive tasks, including attention, concentration, and memory. In this study, the amount and frequency of cocaine use were correlated with the level of neuropsychological impairment. Although this was a small study, it suggests yet another hazard of cocaine use. Future research will focus on the question of whether these changes are reversible with abstinence from cocaine.

Adverse Reactions to Cocaine: Who Is Vulnerable?

Given the widespread popularity of cocaine and the tendency of many individuals to increase both their frequency of use and the dose consumed, one may wonder why the negative effects of the drug described in this chapter are not even more common. One explanation is that there are individual differences in the subjective response to cocaine, which are influenced by both genetic and environmental factors. In addition, the presence or absence of other psychological difficulties, the expectations of the user, and the setting in which the drug is used also influence the response to cocaine. Thus individuals who are preoccupied by stressful life circumstances may be more vulnerable to the dysphoria and/or psychosis that sometimes accompanies cocaine use. Relevant to this issue are the results of laboratory experiments in which administration of amphetamine (a related stimulant drug) to rats previously stressed by fighting or overcrowding appeared to increase the likelihood of overdose and death in these "stressed" animals.

The use of other drugs with cocaine can increase the risk of adverse effects. It is not unusual for someone dependent on cocaine to also use heroin, alcohol, benzodiazepines (drugs like Valium), marijuana, or combinations of these drugs. Because each of these drugs carries its own risk of adverse psychological and physical effects, combining any of them with cocaine increases the likelihood of both medical and psychiatric complications. In particular, the use of alcohol along with cocaine may alter the metabolism of the drug, leading to a breakdown product known as *cocaethylene,* which has been found to be particularly toxic to the heart.

Persons with overt or covert psychiatric disorders appear to be more vulnerable to the disorganizing effects of cocaine, and they may be at greater risk for developing cocaine abuse problems. Our research has shown, for example, that individuals with chronic depression, bipolar disorder (manic-depressive illness), or cyclothymia (a milder form of bipolar disorder) may be particularly vulnerable to the effects of cocaine, which places them at high risk for dependence. The powerful initial effect that cocaine has on some of these individuals may encourage them to use the drug more frequently. Unfortunately, such persons may experience an exacerbation of their mental disorders as a result of their cocaine use. For example, Dr. Robert Post's research (discussed above) showed that depressed patients are just as likely to experience dysphoria (feeling unwell or unhappy) as euphoria during early cocaine use and that they are more likely to experience depression as they increase their dose of the drug.

Individuals with underlying bipolar disorder or cyclothymia are particularly sensitive to the effects of cocaine. In some individuals, manic states may be precipitated or exacerbated by cocaine use. Indeed, some manic or hypomanic individuals report that they use cocaine purposefully to enhance and extend the euphoria they feel as part of their manic episode. Persons with schizophrenia also appear to be more vulnerable to the disorganizing effects of cocaine; some schizophrenic individuals may manifest psychotic thinking or behavior even after relatively low doses of the drug.

Finally, attention-deficit hyperactivity disorder (ADHD), which is characterized by hyperactivity and inattention, has been linked to cocaine use. In Dr. Bruce Rounsaville's aforementioned study of psychiatric illness in cocaine users, one-third of his subjects were found to have a history of ADD. Although this syndrome is characteristically present in childhood and adolescence, a residual form of ADD can persist into adulthood. Persons with ADD frequently have a paradoxical decrease in hyperactivity when given psychostimulants. For this reason, drugs that are similar to amphetamine, such as methylphenidate (Ritalin), are often prescribed as a treatment for ADD. It is possible that some individuals who had ADD as children may be treating residual symptoms of this disorder with cocaine. Support for this hypothesis comes from reports of improvement in cocaine problems when individuals are given appropriate treatment for their ADD.

Although we know that certain groups of individuals have a higher risk for developing cocaine abuse problems, there is no way to predict in advance who will, in fact, suffer adverse effects from the drug. It is precisely this unpredictability that makes cocaine use so hazardous. Cocaine is a very powerful drug that profoundly influences brain function. In the next chapter, we discuss how these alterations of mood and behavior can lead to cocaine dependence.

Chapter 5

Cocaine Dependence

During the worst New England snowstorm in nearly a century, "Richard," a 25-year-old teacher, nearly froze to death because he had sold his car and his only winter coat for a quarter of an ounce of cocaine. Looking back on this decision was frightening, he said,

> Because at the time, I made what seemed like the obvious choice. I just figured, 'Sell the coat, sell the car, get the coke.' I needed the cocaine more.

"Francine," a 23-year-old secretary related an argument she had recently with her fiance:

> I told my boyfriend that I had stopped using cocaine, but he found out from my friends that I was still using when he wasn't around. We've had this fight lots of times, and he usually leaves me alone if I promise him I'll stop using. This time was different. He said he was tired of all my broken promises, and so I was going to have to make a choice—either cocaine or him. I love him, but the choice is clear. I guess it just comes down to the fact that I love coke more than anybody or anything. Sometimes I wonder if I'll regret not getting married to him, but then I remind myself that I don't really want to be with someone who doesn't see how important cocaine is to me.

The American Psychiatric Association (APA), in its *Diagnostic and Statistical Manual of Mental Disorders, Fourth Edition* (DSM-IV), defines *substance dependence* as "a maladaptive pattern of substance use, leading to clinically significant impairment or distress, as manifested by three or more of the following occurring at any time in

71

the same twleve-month period:" (the specific criteria used to make the diagnosis of cocaine dependence in *DSM-IV* are listed in Table 3). The case examples described above highlight a central feature of cocaine dependence (we use the terms *dependence* and *addiction* interchangeably): both Richard and Francine were preoccupied with cocaine. It had become their top priority—above physical well-being, above relationships, perhaps above basic survival instincts.

Table 3. DSM-IV criteria for diagnosing cocaine dependence

Cocaine dependence is a maladaptive pattern of cocaine use, leading to clinically significant impairment or distress, as manifested by three of more of the following occurring at any time in the same twelve-month period:

(1) tolerance, as defined by either of the following:
   (a) need for markedly increased amounts of cocaine to achieve intoxication or desired effect
   (b) markedly diminished effect with continued use of the same amount of cocaine
(2) withdrawal, as manifested by either of the following:
   (a) the characteristic withdrawal syndrome for cocaine
   (b) cocaine (or a closely related substance) is taken to relieve or avoid withdrawal symptoms
(3) cocaine is often taken in larger amounts or over a longer period than was intended
(4) a persistent desire or unsuccessful efforts to cut down or control cocaine use
(5) a great deal of time is spent in activities necessary to obtain cocaine, use cocaine, or recover from its effects
(6) important social, occupational, or recreational activities given up or reduced because of cocaine use
(7) continued cocaine use despite knowledge of having had a persistent or recurrent physical or psychological problem that was likely to have been caused or exacerbated by cocaine (e.g., current cocaine use despite recognition of cocaine-induced depression)

Source. Adapted from American Psychiatric Association: *Diagnostic and Statistical Manual of Mental Disorders, Fourth Edition.* Washington, DC, American Psychiatric Association (in press). Used with permission.

These cases illustrate cocaine dependence in its most severe form, in which users think of little else but the drug and care neither for other people nor themselves.

It is significant to note that the current APA view of dependence (which is echoed in recent definitions by the National Institute on Drug Abuse and the World Health Association) does not distinguish between "physical" and "psychological" dependence. Indeed, the emphasis on the compulsion to use the drug repeatedly represents a departure from older definitions of drug dependence, which required the presence of tolerance (the need for markedly increased drug intake to achieve the desired effect) or physical withdrawal symptoms. This redefinition of dependence was, in part, based on recent experience with cocaine. Because cocaine, unlike heroin or alcohol, does not cause a dramatic withdrawal syndrome, it was formerly considered "nonaddicting." This separation of physical versus psychological dependence was based on the mistaken belief that the avoidance of physical symptoms provides the primary motivation for drug users to continue their habit. Recent clinical experience and brain research (see Chapter 4) have shown otherwise: it is now widely accepted that cocaine can and does cause profound dependence, or addiction.

How does cocaine dependence develop? Who is at risk? In this chapter, we attempt to answer these questions in several ways. First, we describe a variety of theories that have been put forth to explain the etiology of dependence; we then describe the typical course of cocaine dependence; finally, we relate a case history of a young woman who developed profound dependence on cocaine after using the drug "safely" for several years.

Factors Contributing to Cocaine Dependence

Psychological Factors

One theory of cocaine dependence that is frequently espoused by health care professionals and addicted patients themselves is that people who abuse cocaine have an underlying personality weakness, which is characterized by an inability to develop useful strategies for coping with stress. Other characteristics of this "addictive personality" include the tendency to be demanding, selfish, manipulative, and passive aggressive. Addicts are often unable to tolerate even moderate amounts of frustration and frequently cannot understand or empathize with the feelings of others.

One major problem in accepting the validity of the concept of the "addictive personality" is the difficulty in determining the causes of these behaviors. Indeed, many of these traits may be the result of, rather than the cause of, drug use. For people who are forced to "hustle" on the street to support their continued use of an illegal drug, a certain degree of manipulativeness and selfishness may be necessary for their survival. These personality characteristics also reflect the power of addiction. As Richard and Francine articulated so poignantly, the most significant relationship in the addict's life is the one with cocaine. If other relationships interfere with the ability to obtain or use cocaine, then those relationships will suffer. It is therefore easy to see how respect and empathy for others can also suffer.

Are manipulativeness, selfishness, and lack of empathy enduring personality traits in people who abuse drugs, or are they the inevitable result of addiction? No one has clearly answered this question. However, similar personality descriptions have been applied to individuals with alcoholism, and a research project by scientists at Harvard Medical School helped to sort out some of the confusion surrounding the causes and consequences of that disorder. By studying a group of men from their adolescence into their mid-40s, Dr. George Vaillant and his colleagues were able to observe a subgroup of men who developed alcoholism. When the researchers reviewed the personality traits of the alcoholic subgroup that were recorded before the development of alcoholism, they found that the personality characteristics frequently ascribed to individuals in this subgroup—such as dependency, passive aggressiveness, selfishness, and manipulativeness—were noted no more frequently in these individuals than in their nonalcoholic counterparts. Dr. Vaillant and his colleagues therefore concluded that these personality traits (sometimes referred to as the *alcoholic personality*) tend to occur as a *result* of long-term excess drinking, not as an underlying *cause*.

Our research with cocaine-addicted patients similarly suggests that there is no "cocaine personality" underlying the development of cocaine dependence. We recently studied more than 50 cocaine users in treatment and asked them about personality characteristics *before* the onset of their cocaine use. From individual to individual, personality characteristics varied widely—there was no set of traits that these patients had in common.

It therefore appears unlikely that all or even most substance-addicted individuals have an "addictive personality" that underlies or causes their addiction. This does not rule out the possibility that some individuals are vulnerable to developing addictions because they have personality traits that lead them to engage in behaviors associated with substance abuse. Dr. Robert Cloninger of Washington University in St. Louis, Missouri, has found that the personality traits of "novelty seeking" (excitement seeking) and low "harm avoidance" (ignoring risk) may be associated with the development of alcohol problems. In one of his studies, 11-year-old boys with these characteristics developed alcohol problems in early adulthood more often than boys without these personality traits. Dr. Cloninger hypothesized that these traits are at least partially inherited and that they reflect variations in brain chemistry. For example, he speculated that the trait of novelty seeking may be related to greater brain sensitivity to dopamine, which is a neurotransmitter involved in the perception of pleasure and reward. Based on this theory, Dr. Cloninger has suggested that the personality traits of novelty seeking and low harm avoidance would make an individual more vulnerable to cocaine abuse as well, although there are no studies to date that support this supposition.

A second hypothesis, closely related to the "personality weakness" theory of cocaine abuse, is that some individuals abuse drugs to obtain relief from intolerable emotional states, particularly depression, anxiety, and anger. According to this "self-medication" hypothesis of cocaine use, an individual with depression might seek out cocaine to relieve his or her low mood. Sometimes, the initial use of cocaine to medicate these painful feelings is consciously planned by the user. Other times, a serendipitous experience with the drug provides a deep sense of relief from emotional discomfort. In such cases, the individual may wish to repeat the comforting experience until a pattern of long-term use develops.

To test this self-medication hypothesis, we studied more than 400 drug users in treatment and found that most reported using drugs to relieve depressive symptoms. Although most of these patients claimed to experience mood improvement with drug use, some actually reported that chronic drug use worsened their depression. It is possible that the initial euphoria experienced with drug administration (such as with cocaine) may reinforce the belief that the drug is improving mood, even though it is in reality leading to increased depression over time.

A related finding from our research with cocaine users is the presence of a high rate of mood disorders among long-term cocaine users admitted to our hospital unit. Approximately 20% of our cocaine abuse patients concurrently have manic-depressive illness (recurrent mood swings shifting from euphoria to depression), and 15% have a serious depressive disorder. Whether these mood problems existed before the onset of cocaine addiction, however, is difficult to ascertain. Dr. Bruce Rounsaville's study of cocaine-dependent patients (discussed in Chapter 4), which reported an equally high rate of mood disorders, also found that most of these mood disorders appeared to begin after or coincident with the onset of cocaine abuse.

Thus one of the shortcomings of the "self-medication" theory of cocaine use is the fact that the drug's ability to relieve depression is generally short lived; in fact, cocaine use may lead to the *development* of depression in chronic users. Research by Dr. Robert Post at the National Institute of Mental Health (see Chapter 4) has shown, in fact, that cocaine may be more of a mood enhancer than a mood elevator. Many people use cocaine as a "party drug"; they find that cocaine initially heightens the experience of an already good mood. However, these same individuals often avoid cocaine when they are depressed because they find that the drug worsens their already low mood.

Although cocaine initially causes euphoria in many occasional users, most long-term cocaine users experience a mixture of depression, irritability, anxiety, and paranoia while on the drug. Despite these clearly noxious effects of chronic cocaine use on physical and psychological functioning, many long-term users continue to self-administer the drug until forced to discontinue it because of decreased drug availability, social or legal pressure, or medical complications. Clinicians who work with these patients are often at a loss to explain why they continue to use the drug despite its devastating consequences. Part of the explanation may rest in the difference between the actual drug experience and the individual's recollection of that experience. This discrepancy can be partially understood by the concept of state-dependent learning, in which events that occur during episodes of intoxication are poorly recalled once the individual is drug free. Thus cocaine-addicted patients in drug treatment programs often nostalgically recall even nightmarish episodes of intoxication.

State-dependent learning cannot, unfortunately, explain why some people feel compelled to continue using cocaine despite their recognition that it makes them feel worse than when they are drug free. According to one patient,

> I hate what the drug does. It makes me cry, it makes me crazy, it makes me think people are trying to kill me, it makes me turn all the lights off in my house and sit at my window for hours, just waiting for someone to climb down out of the trees so that I can get a gun and shoot him. I'm not like this usually. The drug does all of this to me. I hate what it does, but I love it. I love the looks of it, I love the taste, I love the smell, I love the feel, I love the action—I love it more than I've ever loved anything else in my life.

For such persons, continued cocaine use cannot be ascribed to the relief from unpleasant feelings, as these individuals often report feeling worse on drugs than off them. Some researchers have attempted to explain continued drug use in this group by suggesting that there are some cocaine users whose primary goal is to alter their mood, regardless of the direction of the change; they are simply looking for a new set of feelings. For some individuals who, for example, have suffered at the hands of abusive parents or who have been the victims of chaotic mood swings, the desire to control the timing of their mood changes may be so crucial that the direction of mood change becomes comparatively unimportant.

Biological Factors

It has become increasingly apparent that understanding personality characteristics and inner psychological conflicts does not sufficiently explain the complexities of addictive behavior. Moreover, it is clear that individuals who experience significant psychological difficulties or social, cultural, or economic deprivation do not necessarily seek relief through the abuse of cocaine or other psychoactive drugs. Researchers are beginning to see that vulnerability to drug abuse is not attributable to one factor such as personality, but instead is most likely related to multiple factors, including both environmental and biological influences.

Research to help understand the biological and genetic origins of substance abuse problems has been attempted for many years. Genetic vulnerability to alcoholism has been the most widely studied; vulnerability to drug use, including cocaine, has rarely been studied specifically. One method of investigating the cause of substance abuse problems has been to study the families of alcohol-dependent patients and to design biological research projects to determine whether those who develop substance abuse problems are "biologically programmed" for dependence. For instance, some people may initially respond to alcohol or drugs in a particular way that increases the likelihood of future abuse problems. By examining findings from research that has already been done on other drugs and alcohol, perhaps we can hypothesize about some of the biological factors that may predispose certain individuals to abuse cocaine.

Family studies.   It has long been recognized that alcoholism runs in families; the rate of alcoholism in first-degree relatives of alcoholic individuals is approximately four times that of family members of nonalcoholic individuals. Family studies of cocaine users and other drug-dependent individuals are rare.

However, in one recent study, Dr. Norman Miller and colleagues looked at individuals addicted to cocaine and found a high rate of *alcoholism* in their families. In fact, the rate of alcoholism in first-degree relatives of cocaine users was similar to that seen in the families of alcoholic individuals. These researchers hypothesized that people with cocaine addiction may share some of the same genetic vulnerabilities as people with alcoholism. Although these findings are provocative, they do not tell us whether we are seeing the result of genetically inherited factors or of learned behavior. Brown hair runs in families; so does speaking English. However, the first trait is transmitted biologically, and the other is learned.

One one that researchers try to distinguish between the respective contributions of "nature" and "nurture" is to study the characteristics of twins. The results of such studies support the presence of a genetically inherited vulnerability to the development of alcoholism; the rate of alcoholism in the identical twins of alcoholic people is twice that of fraternal twins. These data suggest that there is probably a genetically inherited vulnerability to alcoholism that is shared more by identical twins, who have the same genetic endowment, than by fraternal twins, who have fewer genes in common. However, the fact that not all identical twins share alcoholism suggests that environmental factors also play a role. Indeed, it can be argued that identical twins often have a significantly different developmental experience from the general population as the result of being twins; this experience may adversely affect health and emotional well-being and promote the development of alcoholism.

Adoption studies, which compare the histories of biological and adoptive families of alcoholic subjects who were adopted at birth, shed even more light on the relative contributions of genetic and environmental factors to the development of alcoholism. In these studies, the presence of alcoholism in a biological parent is the single most reliable predictor of alcoholism in the offspring, regardless of whether the child is adopted by alcoholic or nondrinking parents. In contrast, adoptees born of nonalcoholic biological parents do not themselves develop alcoholism at any greater rate than the general population, even if they are reared by alcoholic adoptive parents. These studies lend considerable weight to the argument that genetic factors are important in the development of alcoholism. There has been one study looking at the development of drug abuse in adopted individuals. Dr. Remi Cadoret and his co-workers at the University of Iowa found that high rates of drug dependence were associated with alcoholism in biological parents. This study suggests that drug abuse, too, has a strong biological component. Furthermore, as shown in the family studies described earlier, Dr. Cadoret's research found that vulnerability to drug and alcohol abuse may come from a common genetic etiology.

It may seem puzzling that a disorder like alcoholism, which involves voluntary behavior (drinking), can be genetically inherited. Several theories have been proposed to explain how this might be the case. Some have suggested that individuals vulnerable to the development of alcoholism may react to alcohol quite differently from those at less risk, even before the development of alcoholism. Some researchers have hypothesized that alcoholic individuals have a dramatic response to their first exposure to drinking. However, research studies comparing the effect of alcohol on alcoholic versus nonalcoholic subjects cannot differentiate whether the different responses in the two populations occur as the result of chronic alcoholism or the different response to alcohol was, indeed, a risk factor for the future development of alcoholism.

A University of California researcher, Dr. Mark Schuckit, developed an ingenious strategy to differentiate the causes of alcoholism from its effects. He studied a group of young men who were sons of alcoholic parents and compared them with men of the same age and educational background who had no family history of alcoholism. Because of their family backgrounds, the first group had a much higher risk for the future development of alcoholism, although none had current drinking problems. Dr. Schuckit felt that if he could detect differences between these two groups he might be able to identify risk factors that preceded alcoholic drinking. The results of the study were striking. Dr. Schuckit found that there were differences between the two groups and that the sons of alcoholic parents exhibited a less dramatic response to alcohol than did the sons of nonalcoholic parents; they were able to perform fine motor tasks more skillfully after drinking and felt less intoxicated.

Other comparative studies of these two groups have shown differences in certain blood hormone levels after drinking. Dr. Schuckit has hypothesized that the impaired ability of some drinkers to determine when they are becoming intoxicated may make it difficult for them to moderate their drinking. Conversely, others who are particularly sensitive to the effects of alcohol may alter their drinking patterns accordingly. For example, some Asians frequently experience flushing, rapid heart rate, abdominal pain, and weakness following relatively small doses of alcohol. These unpleasant effects, which may be caused by a relative lack of one of the enzymes that breaks down alcohol, have been cited as a major factor in the low rate of alcohol abuse in most Asian cultures.

Thus we can see how the variability in the initial response to a drug may place some people at higher risk for future abuse problems. Although this hypothesis has been studied primarily in alcoholic subjects, there is some evidence of a differential response to cocaine as well. In an experiment designed to assess the effect of cocaine on mood, Dr. Richard Resnick and his colleagues at New York Medical College administered 25 milligrams (approximately two lines) of cocaine to a group of regular users of the drug. Twelve subjects received the drug intravenously, and 12 received it intranasally. Although most subjects experienced the drug as pleasant and relaxing, 4 of the intravenous users and 2 of the intranasal users reported dysphoric effects (feeling unwell or unhappy) after the period of euphoria. They described feelings of anxiety, fatigue, and depression and expressed a desire for more cocaine. Therefore, it is possible that cocaine users who "crash" readily may be at risk for developing abuse problems earlier than users who experience less craving for the drug after the euphoria ends.

Biological markers in addictive disorders. Family studies such as those described above demonstrate that there is likely an inherited component to the development of alcoholism. Ultimately, some researchers hope to identify a gene or genes that transmit a susceptibility to developing alcoholism or other addictions. Genes are the biological units of heredity; made up of DNA, they are passed from one generation to the next. In 1990, researchers in Los Angeles thought that they had discovered such a gene; they found that alcoholic parents and their children had a particular form of the gene for dopamine receptors (known as the *D2-adrenergic receptor*). Although this finding is provocative, it has not thus far been replicated by subsequent studies and must therefore still be viewed as speculative.

Another line of inquiry in the search for the causes of addiction has been the attempt to find biological markers that may identify individuals who are at increased risk for the development of one or more of these addictive disorders. These markers may also help researchers locate genes involved in passing vulnerability to addictions from generation to generation. Biological markers may include abnormal physical characteristics or the degree of activity of particular chemicals in the body. Thus, for example, although the accumulated data are thus far inconclusive, there is some evidence that the level of activity of a chemical called *monoamine oxidase (MAO),* which can be measured in the blood, may be decreased in some alcoholic individuals. Moreover, MAO levels appear to be reduced in the relatives of individuals with low MAO activity, particularly in those relatives who are alcoholic themselves. Low MAO activity has also been documented in individuals with schizophrenia, depression, and certain personality traits such as impulsiveness. It is therefore unclear whether low MAO activity is actually a useful marker for alcoholism or whether it is a nonspecific marker of psychopathology.

A second potential marker for alcoholism that has been explored is electroencephalographic (EEG) or brain wave activity. Recordings of EEG activity in alcoholic subjects have shown more high-frequency activity, which characterizes states of decreased arousal, compared with control subjects. This EEG finding has also been found in some studies of sons of alcoholic parents, which raises the possibility that this abnormal brain wave activity is inherited. Furthermore, some researchers have found that even sons of alcoholic parents who are not alcoholic themselves have increased high-frequency activity, which demonstrates that these EEG findings are not merely the result of repetitive alcohol consumption. It has yet to be shown, however, whether having this EEG finding in some way predisposes individuals to the development of alcoholism or it is an incidental finding.

Another group of biological markers that may affect the vulnerability to the subsequent development of drug and alcohol abuse involves the opioid-like compounds (endorphins) that are made in the body. These brain chemicals, which have been identified only in the past decade, appear to exert effects similar to those of opioid (narcotic) drugs. Thus the release of endorphins after a minor injury will help a person be less concerned about the pain just suffered. Some researchers have postulated that certain individuals are born with a deficiency of these substances, thus impairing their capacity to cope with physical or emotional distress. These persons may therefore be more likely to have a dramatic emotional response to opioid drugs such as morphine, heroin, or codeine. According to this theory, their use of opioid drugs fulfills a biological need and, in some respects, corrects a physiological abnormality.

Similar arguments have been advanced to explain the tendency among some people to abuse antianxiety drugs such as diazepam (Valium). These individuals may be congenitally deficient in certain naturally occurring antianxiety compounds, thus theoretically rendering them less able to handle "normal" amounts of anxiety. Using the same reasoning, some investigators have suggested that users of central nervous system stimulants like cocaine, which increase turnover of brain chemicals called *catecholamines,* particularly dopamine and norepinephrine (see Chapter 4), may have an underlying deficiency of catecholamines in their brains, which is at least temporarily relieved by self-administration of these compounds. This relatively low level of brain catecholamines may show up as symptoms of depression.

Social Factors

Although recent advances in pharmacology and brain chemistry research have helped elucidate the mechanism of action of cocaine, biological factors alone cannot explain a behavioral phenomenon as complicated as addiction. It is important to keep in mind that drug abuse occurs within a social context. Thus the environment in which drug taking occurs profoundly influences the nature of the user's behavior. Critical environmental influences include relationships with family, friends, and peers, as well as the individual's role within larger social institutions, including religion, social class, and the legal system.

Drugs as a social lubricant. A number of drug users recount that their initial experiences with drugs like cocaine, alcohol, and marijuana were designed to help them communicate better with others. Indeed, in small quantities these substances decrease inhibitions and at times enable people to express feelings that they would ordinarily keep to themselves. However, with heavier use of these drugs, their facilitating effect on interpersonal communication is lost; people highly intoxicated on marijuana tend to become self-absorbed and somnolent, whereas large amounts of cocaine or alcohol may cause increased aggressiveness and poor judgment.

From the standpoint of peer group interaction, drug use may provide the focus for shared activity. A number of research studies have shown that people who use large amounts of drugs or alcohol tend to cultivate relationships with other heavy drug users. These individuals, who often have little sense of their own identity, find within the drug-using peer group a degree of acceptance, a clear set of behavioral expectations, and approval for continuing their drug-using life-style. Adolescents appear to be particularly vulnerable to this subtle form of peer pressure.

Furthermore, there have been several periods in history during which drug use was the behavioral expression of certain social and cultural values. During the 1960s, for example, the use of lysergic acid diethylamide (LSD) and other hallucinogens took place in the context of a rebellion against traditional middle-class values. The phrase "turn on, tune in, and drop out" suggested that hallucinogen use was one means by which certain groups could separate themselves from what they saw as an unjust society. Although less common than a decade ago, cocaine use today still may represent an expression of financial and social success—of having "made it." According to "Paul," a 28-year-old stockbroker,

> Doing coke alone defeats part of the purpose of it. You do it around certain people to show who you are. You're up and coming, you're one step ahead of the game, and they'd better watch out. People used to join country clubs as a status symbol so that they could talk about it to their friends and co-workers. In our office, people invest in "blow" for the same reason. Unfortunately, it's a damned expensive and damaging way to give people the message that you're hot.

Finally, some individuals become involved with illicit drug use because they are attracted to the deviant life-style that often accompanies such use. For them, the excitement of the illegal activity that is often required to obtain drugs may be as rewarding as the pharmacological effects of the drugs themselves. Others may find that the use of these drugs may facilitate risk taking or engaging in deviant behavior that they have learned to enjoy.

"Eric," a 22-year-old man who had a history of rebellious behavior both within his family and at school, left his small midwestern hometown to go to New York, where his stated goal was to become a heroin addict. "I wanted to get addicted to heroin because I could think of no other behavior which was more proscribed by society." He said that for the initial several months, he did not particularly enjoy the pharmacological experience of intoxication. However, he relished the challenge of stealing to pay for his habit and enjoyed mingling with "the nether world of our society." He eventually became strongly addicted to heroin and cocaine.

Familial factors. Many clinicians and researchers have attempted to determine the possible role of family relationships in the development of substance abuse. For example, it has been noted that although drug users often pursue a life-style that most people would term *deviant*, they frequently remain involved and perhaps overly entangled with their families of origin. A study of heroin addicts, for instance, revealed that 59% of those studied still lived with their mothers or a female blood relative at age 30. Numerous authors have attempted to describe family backgrounds that might predispose children to drug dependence. One of the most frequently described patterns is a combination of overindulgence and overly harsh, arbitrary punishment. These may both be seen in one parent or may reflect a difference between the mother and father. The overprotectiveness may deprive children of experiencing the normal anxieties and frustrations of growing up. Such individuals may therefore be at an increased risk to seek pharmacological relief from unpleasant feelings because of a lack of other coping skills. The harshness of discipline may allow children to be similarly harsh on others in an attempt to rationalize some of the antisocial behaviors that often accompany drug addiction.

Although such theories of addiction are interesting and at times useful, they have never stood the test of rigorous study. There are clearly many individuals raised within similar family constellations who never develop drug problems. Indeed, many individuals who abuse substances have siblings who do not have similar difficulties. Thus merely invoking pathogenic family interactions cannot explain the development of substance use disorders. No scientific research has ever demonstrated a correlation between any particular family setting or early childhood experience with the subsequent development of alcohol or drug abuse. Moreover, the clinical experience of those who work with many substance users and their families reveals much more about their diversity than their similarity.

Sociocultural factors. We have seen the ways in which psychological, biological, and family experiences can influence an individual's drug choice and his or her subsequent pattern of drug use. The social, cultural, religious, and legal values of one's larger society also profoundly affect the use of drugs and alcohol. For example, the Harrison Narcotics Act of 1914, which outlawed cocaine, nearly wiped out the use of a drug that had been enormously popular in America during the previous 25 years. In addition, the values and norms of a particular sector of society can influence the prevalence of drug use within that sector. An example of this is the growing drug use and drug trade among urban adolescents and young adults, especially those involved with gangs.

Cocaine Dependence

Statistics show that from 1990 to 1991 cocaine use began to rise again in the United States. The prevalence of serious cocaine dependence, as evidenced by daily use, also increased, leading to more cocaine-related emergency room visits and more urban violence. Statistics show some other grim facts: the most substantial increases in cocaine use occurred in urban areas, among blacks, among unemployed individuals, and in those under age 35. Several factors have been suggested to explain this phenomenon. The introduction of crack cocaine has made the drug more affordable to those who may not have been able to buy it previously. In addition, urban gangs have taken over much of the sale and distribution of crack, making it widely available in the inner city.

For urban youths facing the stark economic and social realities of the inner city, involvement in the drug culture can seem appealing. The possibilities of legal, gainful employment are limited—currently, almost 20% of black men in this country are unemployed. Furthermore, for individuals who face potential harm or death from widespread street violence, the prospect of being jailed for involvement in illegal drug activity may not be a major deterrent. In some settings, selling or using drugs is not only accepted, it may seem like the only way to make money or to be "somebody." For a select few, drug dealing does lead to riches. Unfortunately, for most, the risks are high, and the profits are low. The threat of imminent violence is ever present, and addiction is a frequent outcome. "Ron," a 28-year-old street seller of cocaine, described how he got into dealing:

> I came across this gang and they needed me around the neighborhood. I wasn't working, so when I saw the money people were making selling rock [crack] it looked good. So I got with them and they showed me a lot of cocaine. It went pretty smooth at first—I was selling it and they paid me $25 off every $150 I sold. I was making about $150 a day. That was the most money I had had in a while. I didn't smoke much myself at first, but seeing so much cocaine gave me ideas. Then I started smoking more. Soon I just took the cash I was making and spent it on rock. It got so I didn't even care about the money; I was working just to get high.

The influence of social setting and peer group acceptance on drug-using behavior is not limited to cocaine. Indeed, the influence of these factors on patterns of drug use was never more powerfully demonstrated than during the Vietnam War, in which it was estimated that one-third of all American combat soldiers between the ages of 17 and 23 used opioids and, in particular, heroin. Approximately half of this group used these drugs regularly. It appears that several factors contributed to this epidemic of heroin use. First, the drugs were easily available; high-quality heroin could be traded for several packs of American cigarettes. Further, heroin could be used without involving street crime, dirty needles (many people used the drug by smoking or intranasally), and high-priced drug dealers. Finally, the shared horror of the Vietnam experience among combat troops led to widespread acceptance within that group of pharmacological self-treatment for anxiety, depression, paranoia, rage, and despair.

The use of heroin among such a large number of American soldiers in Vietnam illustrates a well-recognized trend in the epidemiology of drug abuse—that psychopathology becomes a less important risk factor for the use of a given drug when the use of that drug becomes more normal and accepted within the society. In other words, the use of heroin in Vietnam was not restricted to a few individuals with long-standing emotional disorders. Rather, the combination of drug availability and a high degree of stress led a large number of people who would not ordinarily use heroin to do so. This phenomenon was corroborated by follow-up studies of opioid-dependent troops, showing that less than 10% of that group ever used opioids again after returning to the United States. Moreover, less than 2% of soldiers who were opioid dependent in Vietnam continued to have serious opioid-related problems after their return from Southeast Asia.

These results are markedly different from studies of individuals who become addicted to heroin in their home environment. Many of these individuals experience cycles of addiction, detoxification, and subsequent relapse that often stretch over a period of years. Therefore, the setting in which drug use and addiction occur, drug availability, and the shared values of one's peer group all play important roles in determining the future outcome of an individual's drug use.

Religious and cultural mores may also have a powerful influence on the use of drugs or alcohol in a society. Epidemiological studies, for example, have shown that certain ethnic or religious groups (e.g., Irish Americans and Native Americans) have greater-than-average rates of alcoholism, whereas others (e.g., Asians and Jews) have lower-than-average rates. Several sociocultural factors have been identified as being potentially important influences on drinking patterns within a society. Among those factors felt to correlate with a relatively low rate of alcoholism are 1) drinking with people of the opposite sex, 2) drinking across generational lines (grandparents, parents, and children drinking together), 3) drinking with meals, 4) drinking as part of a religious ceremony or celebration, and 5) belonging to an ethnic, religious, or social group that treats drunkenness with opprobrium. Though it is difficult to draw an exact parallel with cocaine use, a wide range of social values do exert their influence on the person's use of drugs and alcohol.

Behavioral Factors

Another helpful perspective in our understanding of addiction is that of *learning theory*. Two key concepts that represent the cornerstones of learning theory include operant reinforcement and classical conditioning.

Operant reinforcement. *Operant reinforcement* refers to the ability of a particular event or response within the environment to increase the frequency of a specific behavior. A simple example can be seen in training animals. If you wish to teach an animal a particular piece of behavior, you will reward it with food, affection, or some other positive action when it performs that behavior. If the animal continues to perform the desired behavior because it has been given the reward, then the reward is said to be reinforcing. Using this principle, scientists have found that animals can be taught to perform "work," usually in the form of repeatedly pressing a lever, to receive certain psychoactive drugs, including cocaine. Over time, the animal may be required to work harder and harder to continue receiving the drug.

These types of experiments give us a rough approximation of the relative reinforcing properties of various psychoactive drugs. Not surprisingly, animals have been enticed in such experiments to work for opioids, amphetamine, nicotine, barbiturates, phencyclidine (PCP), and alcohol. However, their response to cocaine was dramatic and unparalleled. Under conditions of unlimited access to intravenous cocaine, rhesus monkeys continued to work for cocaine and self-administer the drug until it caused death.

Some behavioral scientists believe that the powerful reinforcing property of cocaine is sufficient to explain continued drug-seeking behavior even in the absence of preexisting psychological problems, poor interpersonal relationships, biological vulnerability, or peer group pressure. These scientists believe that cocaine is such a powerful drug that it can lead to severe addiction in virtually anyone, as long as it is easily available. This belief has led some outspoken advocates of the legalization of marijuana and heroin to express some misgivings about the legalization of cocaine, because it appears that the growing availability of the drug and the concurrent drop in price have led to a large increase in the number of cocaine-related problems in this country.

Classical conditioning and craving.   *Classical conditioning* was first described at the turn of the century by Russian psychologist Ivan Pavlov, who reported this phenomenon after performing experiments with his dog. Pavlov found that when he repeatedly rang a bell while presenting his dog with food, the dog would salivate at the sound of the bell, because it was concurrently receiving food. When Pavlov later rang the bell without presenting the food, the dog continued to salivate because it had mentally paired the bell with the food to such an extent that the ringing of the bell continued to evoke this *conditioned response.* The concept of Pavlovian (classical) conditioning is important in understanding *craving,* which can be defined simply as a very strong desire for drugs.

Craving may manifest primarily as an emotional state, or it may be accompanied by physical symptoms. The desire for drugs tends to increase when drugs are available and diminish when they are not easily attainable. Craving is often stimulated by conditions previously associated with drug-taking activity; these may include psychological or interpersonal stress, being in the presence of former drug-using companions, or entering a neighborhood in which one has previously taken drugs. Increased craving in response to feelings, places, or people associated with previous drug experiences is another example of a classically conditioned response. This type of reaction may at times trigger relapse.

"Lou," a 30-year-old man, was hospitalized for several weeks because of long-term cocaine use. During that time, he engaged in individual psychotherapy, became involved in Narcotics Anonymous, and attended several groups daily, most of them focusing on ways in which cocaine had adversely affected his life. Two days after being discharged to home, he received a telephone call from his drug dealer, who said, "Where have you been? I've been holding an ounce of cocaine for you for weeks." The patient replied, "Great! When can we get together?" He relapsed that day, but later stated emphatically that he had had no desire to take cocaine before talking with his dealer.

Lou's case clearly illustrates the powers of classical conditioning; under conditions of high drug availability, intense craving can be quickly stimulated and may trigger conditioned behavior in an almost automatic way. Under these circumstances, a cocaine user can quickly lose sight of the potentially harmful consequences of his or her actions. Because of such behavioral responses, we recommend that individuals who are trying to stop cocaine avoid former drug-using companions and localities.

Conditioned responses may include physiological changes in addition to psychological reactions. For example, rats that have been previously addicted to opioids will demonstrate signs of withdrawal when placed in an environment in which they have undergone withdrawal in the past. This phenomenon of "conditioned withdrawal" has been observed in humans as well.

"Larry," a 29-year-old man, was hospitalized for the treatment of heroin addiction. After four weeks of treatment, he returned to his former job, which required him to ride the subway past the stop at which he had previously bought his drugs. Each day, when the subway doors opened at this location, the patient experienced enormous craving for heroin, accompanied by tearing, a runny nose, abdominal cramps, and gooseflesh. After the doors closed, his symptoms disappeared, and he went on to work.

Larry experienced symptoms of heroin withdrawal in this locale when the doors were open because this represented a period of high drug availability. In his mind, heroin withdrawal and this particular subway station were as clearly paired as were the bell and food for Pavlov's dog. Thus he experienced increased drug craving in the most hazardous of all circumstances: when drugs were readily available.

A recent study by Dr. Anna Rose Childress and her colleagues at the University of Pennsylvania showed that responses to conditioned stimuli can be altered by mood. These researchers elicited negative mood states such as depression, anxiety, and anger in subjects addicted to opioids through a hypnotic procedure. They found that their subjects who experienced negative mood states were more likely to experience conditioned symptoms of opioid withdrawal when presented with drug cues. Subjects who felt euphoric rather than depressed, anxious, or angry responded less to drug-related cues. Thus the degree of response to conditioned stimuli can be influenced by the mood of the respondent. Perhaps other factors will also be discovered that decrease the strength of conditioned responses. This information could potentially be very useful in the treatment of cocaine addiction.

Many substance users find that as their addiction develops, they become "hooked" on conditioned stimuli: drug paraphernalia, needles, razor blades, mirrors, "coke spoons," stealing, scheming, and procuring drugs. Indeed, there are some individuals, known as "needle freaks," who will inject themselves with water if there are no drugs available, because they derive pleasure merely from the experience of injection itself.

Two activities that seem to coexist frequently with cocaine use are gambling and sex. For example, studies of cocaine-dependent patients have revealed a prevalence rate of pathological gambling ranging from 15% to 30%—10 to 20 times the estimated rate in the general population. Dr. Arnold Washton has also reported the frequent coexistence of compulsive sexual behaviors and cocaine use. A subgroup of cocaine users frequently engage in sexual fantasy or experimental sexual behavior while intoxicated and may eventually come to rely on the drug to function sexually at all. For some users, these components of the addictive life-style become as important as the pharmacological activity of the drugs and may act as triggers for relapse if not identified and addressed appropriately. When these conditioned stimuli constitute an important part of an individual's addiction, altering the pattern of drug dependence can be very difficult without making major changes in life-style at the same time.

The Course of Cocaine Dependence

Not all cocaine users develop dependence. Rather, the use of cocaine occurs along a continuum from one-time experimentation to severe addiction. Cocaine use causes very few problems for some individuals, creates temporary difficulties in others, and ruins or ends the lives of still others. This unpredictability is one of the most dangerous properties of cocaine. Smoking cocaine freebase or crack, however, seems to lead to addiction more rapidly and more often than using cocaine in other forms. This is most likely due to the intensity and rapid onset of the "high" (see Chapter 2). Crack has acquired a dangerous reputation that frightens away many potential users who have not used cocaine before. Unfortunately, many crack users start using cocaine intranasally—a method of cocaine use still considered to be "safe" by some. Once using cocaine intranasally, an individual may be willing to take greater risks, including trying crack. The story of "Ellen" at the end of this chapter is an example of this phenomenon.

Dr. Robert L. DuPont, former director of the National Institute on Drug Abuse, has called "experimentation and first time use" the first of four stages of the drug dependence syndrome, with the latter three stages being "occasional use," "regular use," and "dependence." Experimentation with cocaine is often disappointing; many first-time users wonder why cocaine is so popular, and they frequently feel that the drug is overrated and overpriced. Some users will stop at this stage simply because they had only wanted to try the drug once; others will cease cocaine use because of their disappointment in its effects. Some who have had an unremarkable experience, however, will be convinced by their friends to try the drug several more times to get used to it. Many patients have told us that they did not truly enjoy cocaine until they had used it sporadically for weeks or even months. Some of these individuals had incorrectly believed that their initial lack of response to cocaine would protect them against future difficulties with the drug. Unfortunately, they were mistaken, because the course of cocaine dependence is highly variable. Although some people realize soon after exposure to cocaine that they cannot stop using the drug, others may use cocaine with few adverse consequences for months or years before they become dependent.

Unlike the group mentioned above, there is a small but significant group of individuals who are profoundly affected by their first dose of cocaine; some develop a craving for the drug after using it just once. "Andy," a 37-year-old man, described this experience:

> I was at a party with a group of friends, and at 11 o'clock this guy brings out some cocaine. I had never seen the stuff before, and I had never been much of a drug user. Maybe I'd smoked a few joints here and there, but nothing serious. I never even drank heavily. But I was having a good time and was feeling rather adventurous that night, so I decided that I would try some coke. A bunch of us sat around and snorted the stuff, and after two little lines of this drug, it was all over. I've never felt anything like it in my life. From that moment on, I knew that cocaine was the drug for me. It was as if I had been born to use cocaine. I felt that I could talk to people, like I was the life of the party, that I could think more clearly, that I was in control. In one minute, I went from being an ordinary, shy, straight-arrow guy to being a king. So far, so good. The problem started a couple of hours later, when the party broke up. Everybody else went home smiling and talking about what a great time they had had. All I could think about was how to find more cocaine. I swear, in two hours I was well on my way to becoming an addict.

Although Andy's story is dramatic and unusual, it is not unique. The progression from experimentation to dependence can take place over an extended period of time or may occur quite quickly. For Andy and others like him who have a dramatic response to cocaine, dependence is not a foregone conclusion. Some people are frightened by their dramatic reaction to the drug and therefore avoid it, lest they become dependent. Others continue to use the drug on occasion, without progressing to further stages of cocaine abuse, because they set strict guidelines for their drug use and never violate them. However, it is quite important to realize that the progression to drug dependence is typically filled with broken promises that are made to oneself, friends, and family members.

How Dependence Develops

Dependence on cocaine may occur under a variety of circumstances and may develop in a matter of days or over a period of several years. However, there are certain aspects of the addictive process that are nearly universal. One major feature of the disorder is the continued use of the drug despite its adverse consequences. Many people in our society develop *temporary* problems as a result of alcohol or drug use. However, most people who have such reactions alter their future behavior to avoid experiencing the problem again. Thus an individual who realizes that he or she is intoxicated when driving home from a restaurant may refrain from drinking and driving in the future. Addicted individuals, however, do not react in this way, because they frequently fail to see the connection between their drug use and their difficulties.

This inability to appreciate the destructive effects of drug use is generally referred to as *denial.* Indeed, addiction has often been called "a disease of denial." Denial becomes an integral part of the addictive process because most addicted people care more about their drugs than about anything or anyone else in their lives. The first goal of any drug-dependent person is obtaining and using drugs; everything else on his or her list of priorities is tied for a distant second. Relationships, work, money, and physical health become secondary considerations.

Drug dependence changes a person's values, so that things that were formerly important no longer seem to matter. This was demonstrated quite dramatically in the case of "Frank," a 29-year-old cocaine user, who was referred to one of us (Dr. Weiss) for a consultation:

Dr. Weiss: How much cocaine do you use in a week?

Frank: About three grams.

Dr. Weiss: So you're spending about $300 a week. How much money do you take home from work?

Frank: Maybe $350.

Dr. Weiss: That doesn't leave you much money for anything else.

Frank: That's right.

Dr. Weiss: What do you do for rent and food money?

Frank: I eat enough to get by, but I'm probably going to be evicted soon, since I can't pay the rent.

Dr. Weiss: So you spend your rent money on cocaine?

Frank: I keep telling myself when I get my paycheck that I'm going to drive directly to my landlord's place and pay him off. The problem is that I always make a little coke stop on the way, and I don't have any money by the time I get to my landlord's place. I keep telling myself that something will work out, but I'm not sure how.

Frank is caught in the throes of cocaine dependence; his values have been altered so severely that the acquisition of cocaine has assumed greater importance in his life than food and shelter. When drugs become this important to an individual, then he physically and psychologically protects himself against anything that might interfere with the continuation of his drug use. For the addict, this generally means protecting himself vigilantly against facing reality, because heavy drug use invariably causes problems. Through the use of denial and rationalization, the cocaine-dependent person can blame his or her problems on other people, on bad luck, and on anyone or anything except his or her drug use.

Fortunately, repeated confrontation with reality may interfere with the denial process, and many long-term cocaine users eventually come to realize the damage that the drug is causing them. However, even addicted users whose denial breaks down may have difficulty stopping their drug use. If a heavy user makes a sincere but unsuccessful effort to stop using cocaine, panic may set in. "Emily," a 31-year-old divorced accountant and mother of a 2-year-old son, described this phenomenon:

> My family was telling me for a long time that my cocaine use was a problem, that I would lose my job, and that my son was being neglected. They told me to stop using, but I didn't think they knew what they were talking about. Even after I got fired from my job, I still thought things were generally going well. I also sincerely felt for a long time that I could stop using the drug anytime I set my mind to it. Then two months ago, my parents told me they were petitioning for custody of my son. They said there was no way I could be a good mother while I was high all the time. My son means everything to me, so I decided I would really try to stop using cocaine. I was able to stop for only four days. Then I found out that I was pregnant again. At that point, I knew things had gone too far. My life was a mess because of cocaine, but I couldn't stop using the drug. I felt scared all of the time, since I knew I would lose my son and my baby if I kept using. But instead of stopping, I just used more cocaine. At least when I was high I didn't think about what was happening to me, my son, and my new baby. But after I used, I would start feeling guilty all over again. I was convinced that my baby would turn out to be deformed because of all the cocaine I was using. Finally, I could see no way out. I felt so hopeless that I thought about killing myself. Fortunately, my family knew how desperate I was and got me into treatment.

Emily's poignant and frightening account illustrates the desperation of the addicted user, the guilt that often ensues, and the inability to use that guilt in a constructive manner to alter behavior. Rather than stopping the cocaine use to lessen her guilt, her sense of powerlessness over her addiction led her to use even more heavily to escape her guilty feelings.

Thus we often see a progression from the initial euphoria of cocaine use to a stage of temporary drug-related difficulties; these problems may lead to either a reduction of or a complete end to cocaine use or to denial of the true cause of the difficulties. If denial occurs, the drug-related problems may be come more intense and frequent; this may eventually lead to a reduction in the level of denial, although it may be too late at this point to easily turn the drug problem around. Some individuals will still be able to stop at this point, whereas others will attempt to stop drug use and fail. These individuals often enter a period of rapidly increasing drug use, borne out of panic, desperation, hopelessness, and a feverish attempt to dispel these feelings.

In describing the course of addiction, we have stressed the potential importance of *denial* in the worsening of the disorder. What exactly do we mean by this term? More important, how can we understand it? Many family members, friends, colleagues, and health care professionals working with substance users have been amazed at the capacity of these individuals to seemingly ignore the role of their drug taking in the creation of their difficulties. "Bill," a 34-year-old cocaine-addicted user who had been drug free for three years, explained his own denial quite well:

I had been an occasional coke user, maybe once or twice a month, for a couple of years before I started to get into it pretty heavily. I had just started making some money with a business that I owned, and I was running in some pretty fast circles. Offering cocaine was just a way of saying hello to some of those people. Deep in my heart, I knew I had a problem a few months later when I realized that my new-found money and a lot of my savings were all going for drugs.

For example, there was the day when I went out to buy my two-year-old son a birthday present, and I came home with an empty pocket and a sore nose. My wife confronted me, and I made this grandstand play. I took out two Bibles that we had in the house and put my right hand on them and swore to God that I had not been using cocaine. I made up this elaborate story about having been unable to find our son the perfect present, and I said that I would go out the next day to another store to find it. As I was telling this story, I knew perfectly well that I was lying, but it seemed to make sense. In that particular frame of mind, I hadn't done anything wrong. I was still high, and the drug reinforced my denial, because it made me feel so good. I felt that this drug was saying to me, "The hell with her, Bill. Just get her off your back. I can make you feel better."

At that point, I truly believed that I needed the drug more than anything else in the world. I was reacting as if I had a life-threatening illness and that the cure for it was to take as much cocaine as I could get, as often as possible. With that as my assumption, lying meant nothing to me, people meant nothing to me, my work meant nothing to me, my beautiful little boy meant nothing to me. What I didn't realize at the time—but what is perfectly clear to me now—is that I did have an illness. But the illness was caused by cocaine, rather than being cured by it. I think that I was denying the reality of what was going on because I felt so bad without cocaine, and because I felt so powerless over that drug, that I couldn't bear thinking about life without it. I had to try to convince myself that cocaine was not my problem, because admitting the truth would force me to either accept being an addict or try to give up the drug. Both choices were totally intolerable.

As illustrated in Bill's story, the progression of dependence is generally accompanied by a gradual alteration of a person's expectations of himself or herself to fit this behavior. This process occurs in all of us at times, and it can be quite adaptive, such as during aging. As we grow older, we realize that we are physically less able to perform certain feats that we used to be able to accomplish during our youth. It is a sign of maturity to accept this fact and to change our expectations of ourselves accordingly. This same phenomenon also occurs in addicted users, but it occurs in response to their addictive disorder instead of as the result of normal development. As their behavior—lying, stealing, or cheating—deviates from their former goals for themselves, their expectations change; they may rationalize these acts as if they are an unavoidable by-product of their hostile environment. Frequently, the first step in recovery from cocaine dependence is the acceptance that this type of behavior is not necessary, but is a symptom of an illness.

The following interview illustrates the use of denial by a 48-year-old executive, "Jim," who was brought by his wife to see one of us (Dr. Weiss) for a consultation. Jim's wife had complained that he was jeopardizing his formerly successful business with erratic decisions and poor management skills; he was irritable and moody, and he had spent $7,000 on cocaine during the previous month. When Jim was interviewed, however, he seemed rather unconcerned by the comments his wife had made, and he shrugged off their importance:

Dr. Weiss: Was your wife accurate when she said that your business is in trouble?

Jim: She's exaggerating. All businesses have their ups and downs.

Dr. Weiss: I'm sure that's true. However, it's my impression that your business had had only "up" periods for a long time, but that it hasn't been thriving lately.

Jim: I don't know what the problem is.

Dr. Weiss: Have you missed many days at work recently?

Jim: Yes, but I can afford to, since I own the business. Nobody checks up on me.

Dr. Weiss: It sounds like that's precisely the problem. When you don't go to work, the company stays open, but it doesn't do very well.

Jim: My employees are well trained. They can run the company without me.

Dr. Weiss: But that's not happening.

Jim: Then there's something wrong with them. I'll have to look into it.

Dr. Weiss: It sounds as if there's something wrong with you, but you don't want to look into it.

Jim: Now you're on my case. I don't know why you listen to everything my wife says.

Dr. Weiss: How many days of work did you miss in the past two months?

Jim: A couple.

Dr. Weiss: Are you saying that you missed only two days of work?

Jim: Maybe a few.
Dr. Weiss: Only three or four days?
Jim: Maybe a little more.
Dr. Weiss: Ten? Fifteen?
Jim: Maybe somewhere in there.
Dr. Weiss: Twenty?
Jim: Fifteen.
Dr. Weiss: All because of cocaine?
Jim: No.
Dr. Weiss: How many were because of cocaine?
Jim: Less than 15.
Dr. Weiss: Fourteen? Thirteen?
Jim: Maybe 13.
Dr. Weiss: So you missed 13 days of work in the past two months because of cocaine. That's almost 2 days a week.
Jim: That sounds like a lot, but it's no big deal. Like I say, the company can run itself.
Dr. Weiss: How long have you been using cocaine?
Jim: About three years.
Dr. Weiss: Did you ever use drugs or alcohol before that in any kind of quantity?
Jim: No.
Dr. Weiss: Then let's think back five years. Five years ago, if you had imagined yourself missing over a third of your workdays because of a drug, and if you had imagined yourself spending the equivalent of $84,000 a year on that same drug, and if you saw your once-successful business collapsing all around you, wouldn't you have thought that that was indicative of a pretty serious problem?
Jim: Yes, I would have.
Dr. Weiss: So what's different now?
Jim: I guess I just don't want to think about it.

Sometimes, even in the heaviest phase of denial, individuals are able to recognize their drug problem when they mentally take themselves out of their present context. It is important to realize that for most cocaine users, the lies, the manipulation, and the rest of the noxious behavior patterns have occurred as a result of their drug use. Many of these individuals had very strong moral convictions before their use of drugs, and they maintain these moral convictions despite the fact that they constantly break them. The process of chipping away at denial often consists of reuniting cocaine users with their own badly eroded sense of values.

One Cocaine User's Story: "Ellen"

The following case history illustrates some of the typical characteristics that are seen frequently in the course of cocaine addiction. These include

1. The initial feelings of power and invincibility caused by cocaine
2. The gradual reliance on cocaine to produce these good feelings and the increasing intolerance of frustration and pain
3. The use of other drugs to offset the unwanted effects of cocaine, such as insomnia
4. A gradual change in life priorities, so that cocaine acquisition and use become a person's most important activities
5. The loss of money and other valuables to pay for the drug
6. Impaired work performance due to drug use
7. Increasing lies and manipulative behavior to maintain cocaine use (this kind of behavior may lead to the alienation of family and friends)
8. Engaging in increasingly dangerous criminal activity to support one's habit
9. Becoming a "coke whore": establishing and maintaining relationships (often, but not necessarily, sexual) for the purpose of acquiring cocaine

The remainder of this chapter is presented in the words of one such cocaine addict, whom we will call "Ellen."

Experimentation and Occasional Use

I first tried cocaine when I was 19 years old. I was hanging out with the guys in my neighborhood and they had some coke. At the time I was afraid, but they convinced me that it would be okay if I tried it with them because they would take care of me if anything bad happened. So I went to one of the guys' house and did two lines, and nothing really happened to me. I didn't get high at all. So they said, "See, it's not that bad, nothing's going to happen to you." So I continued to do more. I wanted to do more at that point to see what would happen to me when it did affect me. Once I realized that I wasn't going to go crazy, I felt less scared and more curious. I'm not sure what I was looking for, exactly, but I think I was hoping for something like pot, but with a little stronger kick. I had smoked pot for three years, and I wanted to get a little bit higher. Pills scared me, for some reason, so I guess that's how I got into coke.

The coke high was a totally different feeling for me, though nothing like pot at all. The first few times I tried it, I felt that I was much more aware of what was going on. One of the first times I tried it, it was snowing; I went outside after I had done it and I was much more aware of the trees and what color everything was. The snow looked so much whiter. It seemed to make me more aware of things, and it made me feel indestructible. Nobody could bother me when I was doing coke. It was as if I was on top of the world. No other drug has ever made me feel like that.

Regular Use

Within a few months, I was getting into coke pretty regularly, and I really felt like Superwoman. I really believed that nothing and no-body could bother me. Here I was, involved with all these very cool people and this very cool drug, and that made me feel kind of special. But the cocaine made me feel like I had a protective bubble around me. I was indestructible: nobody could hurt me physically, emotionally, or with words. In my mind, I could take care of everything. I could bother everybody else, but nobody could bother me.

103

At that point I did coke mostly at night, before going out to a club or dancing. I wasn't spending too much at this point. I'd usually buy a quarter of a gram for $25, or I'd split a half gram with a girlfriend or two. A quarter of a gram was only good for about 10 lines, but it would last me a weekend. I'd go out on a Friday night, do two lines and leave the rest in my apartment, go to a club, have a few drinks, party, hang out, go back to my apartment, wake up on a Saturday morning and maybe do a line, go to the beach all day if it was summertime, and then come back and do the rest of the coke on Saturday night before I went out.

I can't say the drug hurt my love life at that point. Hell, I had good sex when I did coke. I liked it. Not only that, but a lot of times I'd see a guy I wanted to meet. If I had a half gram of coke, I could have him in my apartment with me just like that. I mean, I'd go to a club, and I'd be a little bit buzzed, and I'd have a half gram of coke with me and I'd see a really good looking guy and I'd just walk up to him because I was Superwoman. Since I had already done a few lines, I was high enough to believe that no one was going to reject me. If anyone did, I'd think, "Well, the hell with you, I don't want you anyway." All that was rationalizing. So I would just walk up to a guy, and I would say, "Hi, do you want to do some lines?" It was just an easy way to meet somebody, not only sexually, but just if I didn't want to be alone.

Problem Use

As time went on, I started using cocaine in the morning, before work, during breaks at work, and sometimes right in the middle of my office if I was alone for a few minutes. I thought that was cool because I didn't get caught. Also when I did coke I felt the euphoria that told me I would never get caught.

The first behavior that should have signaled to me that I was in trouble came when I started selling my jewelry. I wasn't making a lot of money, and I couldn't afford to buy coke because by this time I was going through half a gram on the weekends. Sometimes I'd even use half a gram on the weekend and a quarter of a gram during the week. So, piece by piece, I started selling my jewelry. My grandfather had been a fine jewelry maker, and he had given me this beautiful collection of rings, necklaces, and bracelets that had always had tremendous sentimental value to me. I knew when I was selling it that I was never going to get it back, but I thought that having one less ring wasn't as important as having more friends. Now I was attracting false "friends" from turning people on, and these people weren't going to come around me if I didn't have any drugs. So I said to myself, "I have lots of jewelry. I'm not going to miss one piece, and I'm going to have friends all weekend long." Then I sold the next one and then the next one, and I kept telling myself the same thing. When I sold my first piece of jewelry, I was probably spending $80 a week on cocaine for myself, and I was turning a lot of other people on. But I swear, I didn't think anything was wrong. I thought that was just the way it was supposed to be.

My performance at my job was going straight downhill; I'd be up till four or five o'clock in the morning snorting coke, and maybe by six o'clock my heart would stop pounding and I could fall asleep. When all the "normal" people were getting up to go to work, I was sleeping off the drug high from the night before. So I missed a lot of work. But in my head, I said to myself, "Well, you're new at this job, and you're living downtown, where there's a lot of things to do besides work." I really thought that this was all happening just because I was in a new job, and that once I got used to it, I'd get into a healthy pattern and everything would all be okay.

It was around this time that the lying and manipulating started, too. One day, my mother asked me why I never wore my jewelry anymore. I had to lie. I told her that someone had broken into my apartment. I said, "Ma, I came home one day and a necklace was gone; you know the creeps that live in the city." The incredible thing was that the story came out so easily, so naturally, I think I believed it myself. I know now that I was using denial pure and simple and that I blamed my problems on everything and everyone except for myself and cocaine. I was able to deceive myself so easily because I felt that I had to have the drug. I think that cocaine itself also gave me false feelings. I was starting to do coke every day at this point, Monday through Friday, a line here, a line there, and then 10 or 15 lines, sometimes 20 lines on the weekend. I think that the cocaine along with the pot and the alcohol, which "evened me out," gave me false feelings. When I got high, I always felt that I was okay, that there was nothing to worry about.

Dependence

I'd now reached a point where I didn't have many options if I wanted to keep using coke: I could deal, I could steal, or I could sell myself. Before I was through, I did all three. I started with dealing. One of the guys who sold me coke was a big time Valium dealer, and he wanted someone else to make his deliveries for him. I knew that I looked innocent enough, so I figured that the odds of my getting arrested were pretty low. And I couldn't argue with the pay: a half gram of coke per delivery. So I thought I was on top of the world. I was making an average of two deliveries a day and snorting a gram of coke every day without spending a penny. The dealing also gave me a sense of power. People needed me to get their high. If someone was really wasted on coke and he wanted to come down with Valium, he had to rely on me. It was as if I was controlling everything that was going on.

As that year went on, I started dealing coke, too, at first for this guy, then for myself. He would give me an eighth of an ounce [just more than three 3 grams], and I would take it back to my apartment and lock the door, because the coke was starting to make me paranoid at this point. Then I'd try a line to figure out how good it was. Even though I wasn't an expert, I thought I was. Depending on how pure I thought the coke was, I would cut it. A lot of times, especially toward the end of that year, I would keep half for myself, cut the other half, and sell it. I'd give him the money for the eighth of an ounce and I'd get a free gram and a half. That, of course, would be gone in about two hours. I was using two or three grams each weekend night, and about a gram and a half every weeknight. At this point, I never missed a night. And I could keep on working because I had access to enough Valium to get to sleep every night; usually two or three pills would do the trick.

As far as I was concerned, all of this was great. Then one morning, at about eight o'clock, after having slept for only about one hour, this guy that I was in partnership with knocked at my door, and he was out of his mind. I didn't know what was wrong with him. He came into my apartment, ripped it apart, and beat me up. He cracked a glass jar over my head, punched me in the face, and I didn't know why he was flipping out. I found out the next day that he was smoking crack. Because of the way my mind was working, something attracted me to it. I wanted something that was that powerful. Remember, I was Superwoman, and I wasn't about to get so crazy. But I wanted what he had.

Soon afterwards, my connection with this guy ended because he found another girl. But by that time I was spending so much money on coke that I needed some way to con people into giving me coke. With men it was easy; if I had sex, I'd get it. I slept with everybody and his brother because I'd always get more coke. I was what they call a "coke whore." Everybody knew it, but I didn't care. I was sleeping with guys that I never would have looked at twice. I can't even remember some of the guys that I went to bed with. But as long as they had coke, I thought it was wonderful. At the time, I was really convinced that most of these guys were madly in love with me. I did the drugs and I had the euphoria, so I believed that they really thought I was great.

One guy I slept with was a major dealer named "Ray." He had a reputation as the biggest coke fiend around. Of course I was madly in love with him, because he gave me all the coke I wanted and I never had to pay for it. He left town because of legal trouble after a few months, and I met this other guy named "Bill." Same story—I came on to him just to get free coke, and he eventually turned me on to crack. The first time I ever smoked crack, I did one hit and just got a little high, and I left the room disappointed. Later on that night, I did two more hits of crack and that was it. It took me three hits to be totally into it. It was so much better than snorting lines. It was like a lush, mellow high. After I took a hit of crack, I'd just lie back on the couch and close my eyes. My heart didn't beat fast, at least not at the beginning. It was great. When I snorted coke, my nose was either runny or stuffy and it would drip down my throat and I'd feel my heart beating. None of that happened when I first smoked crack.

I smoked crack for about a year, and after two months I was physically, emotionally, and psychologically addicted to it. I had a love-hate relationship with cocaine at this point. I loved doing it and I hated coming down. When I started using crack and there was no more Valium, I literally flipped out when the coke was gone. I couldn't fall asleep, and I would throw things around in my apartment, and I would go up and down on the elevator in the apartment building. I would call people at four or five o'clock in the morning looking for more crack. At that point I started getting into over-the-counter sleeping pills. At four o'clock in the morning, totally high, I would get in my car, drive to an all-night store, buy a bottle of Sominex, go back to my room, and take all 16 pills in the bottle. Two hours later, I would fall asleep; the pills would finally hit me the next day when I'd wake up incredibly sick.

When the relationship with Bill ended, I was in big money trouble. After a month, I owed one coke dealer $3,000 and I had no way to come up with the money. The problem was that dealers knew me, so they would "front" me the coke, meaning that they'd give me the coke with the understanding that I'd pay them later. That only happens when a dealer trusts you, and I had a good rapport with one dealer. I had bought coke from him for four or five months and I always paid, so he eventually started fronting me some crack if I would give him $20 toward it the next day. The thing about coke, though, is that after you get it fronted, it's gone in an hour and you don't want to pay for it the next day. By then, all you want is another hit and you don't even know how you're going to pay for the cocaine you just used. I tried to squeeze a lot of people out of money I owed, and I "borrowed" it from everyone I could, with no intention of paying it back, thinking that I needed the money more than they did. That kind of thinking made all the sense in the world at the time.

Eventually, nobody would give me money, and this dealer was threatening me. I asked this one really sleazy guy for money, and he said that he couldn't lend me the money, but he would have a girlfriend of his give me a call. Anyway, she introduced me to a prostitution ring. I'd sleep with these out-of-town businessmen for $100 and all the cocaine I wanted. At the time, I thought of myself as a high-class call girl. I had all these wonderful words for it, but the bottom line was that I was a hooker. It really started out because I wanted to pay off my debts, but when I would get to the hotel, these guys would turn me on with coke, and in 15 minutes I would be gone with $100 in my hot little hands. But instead of going back to pay the person that I owed, who was threatening to break my legs, I was so addicted from doing that coke with the businessman that I would go back and buy more from somebody else. While I was doing all of this, for five or six months, I knew what I was doing, but somehow I managed to rationalize to myself that I wasn't doing anything wrong. Even though it was totally against all the morals and values that I had been raised with, I just pretended that I was in a fantasyland, like in Alice in Wonderland. I pretended that these were guys that I knew, and that I wanted to go to bed with these guys. I pretended that everything was going to be okay.

I was fired from my job that year. At the end of that year, almost everyone I knew got arrested and I was hiding out from the police with some of the men who paid me to be with them. At this point I weighed 100 pounds. I'm 5'8", so at 100 pounds I was a mess. None of my clothes fit me. I wasn't taking showers. I wasn't going out. I was totally isolating myself in my apartment. I was totally paranoid. People would knock at the door, and I would hide under the covers. If the phone rang, I'd jump. I'd hide in the bathroom. I didn't see anybody. My family and friends would say to me that something was wrong, that they were afraid I was having a problem with cocaine. They offered to help, but I'd say, "No, nothing's wrong, I'm fine." I wanted people off my back.

I knew at this point, after I'd been a prostitute, that I had a problem. And I knew the problem was cocaine. I just wanted people off my back. There was a part of me that still wanted to believe that I could do it socially, that I could stop on my own. I'd quit tomorrow. I quit a hundred thousand times. There was a little part of me that wanted to think I could do it, but my gut feeling was, "You're never going to do it, Ellen. You're going to die doing coke." Then you know what I'd think? This is really perverted. I thought that I'd die happy, as if I was happy. I was so miserable. Coke wasn't getting me high at all anymore. I was so paranoid, I used to hear cars drive up and think they were the police. I'd drive on the streets and I'd always be looking out of my windows and mirrors. I always thought the cops were after me. I always thought people were talking about me. I thought people that I owed money to were all getting together to hire a hit man to kill me. I was too paranoid to go into supermarkets. I couldn't go food shopping. I couldn't go into a department store. I always thought people were looking at me. I thought the security people knew I did coke. Everywhere I went I thought people knew by looking at me, that they could tell. I just felt that everybody was after me.

When I smoked a lot of crack, sometimes I would have trouble catching my breath for a few seconds. One day, though, I couldn't catch my breath for what seemed like an eternity. I was panting and coughing—I thought I was going to die. I couldn't even talk enough to call someone for help. Finally, I was able to breathe again, but that flipped me out. Around that time I really thought I should just kill myself. I was in so much trouble with money, so many people were after me, and it seemed like I couldn't stop doing coke. I couldn't buy it anymore from anybody. I just started stealing it from a couple of coke dealers I went out with, and when they found out it was as if everybody was after me.

At this point, I thought, "To hell with it," and I bought three bottles of sleeping pills and took them all. I really wanted this nightmare to end. But before I started to go to sleep, I got scared and got myself to an emergency room. They pumped my stomach and did a blood test that was heavily positive for cocaine. They told me that if I didn't sign into a drug treatment program voluntarily, they'd hospitalize me against my will. Thank God someone took over for me, because I was heading for disaster. That was the last day that I ever used any drug or alcohol. I have been straight for two years now, I'm engaged to be married, I've got a good job, I've got good relationships with my friends and my family, and I can honestly say that I'm a very happy person.

Chapter 6

Cocaine and the Family

Happy families are all alike; every unhappy family is unhappy in its own way.

—Leo Tolstoy

When 21-year-old "Tom" ran out of money after a cocaine binge, he asked his parents to drive him to New York City to replenish his supply. When they demurred, he threatened to rob a gas station to finance his habit. Tom's parents never found out whether he would have carried out his threat, because they gave in to his request. This scenario was repeated on numerous occasions, always with the same result. Tom's parents ultimately sold their home to continue supporting their son's habit. His mother said, "Whenever I thought of not giving in to him, I imagined him in a shoot-out with the police and I pictured Tom dead. No matter what, I couldn't let that happen to my boy."

"Larry," a 32-year-old man, regularly visited prostitutes when using cocaine. His wife had known of his cocaine use and his extramarital affairs for several years, and she had begged him to stop. Shortly after he entered treatment, Larry's wife informed him that she was leaving because of his drug use. Larry responded by saying, "She always says this after she finds out about one of my flings. She'll get over it in a few weeks if I can keep my nose clean. I never worry about her leaving me."

"Martha," a 36-year-old woman, had used cocaine heavily for three years. Her moods fluctuated rapidly, and she drank heavily in an attempt to "balance out" some of the stimulant effects of cocaine. Her 14-year-old daughter, a former honor-roll student, had recently become truant, started drinking, become promiscuous, and begun experiencing bouts of severe depression.

Cocaine abuse does not occur in a vacuum. For every cocaine user, there is a family that usually suffers greatly. Although the specific behaviors associated with cocaine abuse vary from individual to individual, certain common events wreak havoc on the families of cocaine users.

1. Cocaine users frequently lie about their whereabouts and their drug use, so that family members can rarely believe anything they say.
2. Cocaine users often neglect their usual responsibilities, such as paying bills, remembering appointments, or going to work on time.
3. Cocaine users may deplete their family's finances. Indeed, the financial problems may become so serious that they will resort to drug dealing, burglary, borrowing from loan sharks, or stealing from the family. It is not an uncommon experience for a cocaine user to support his or her habit by pawning wedding rings, family heirlooms, and other irreplaceable items of high sentimental and often low financial worth. Some individuals even resort to stealing their children's savings to support their habits.
4. Cocaine users display rapid mood shifts; they may become quite paranoid, believing that individuals around them are plotting against them. The paranoia, which is frequently accompanied by irritability, impulsiveness, and explosiveness, may lead to verbal or physical attacks on family members.
5. Because cocaine is often associated with sexuality, it may initially be used in the context of extramarital affairs, thus making the drug use even more distressing to the spouse. In addition, long-term cocaine use frequently causes sexual dysfunction, which can also place great stress on a marriage.

It is easy to see how this pattern of behavioral disturbances can create enormous difficulties within a family. In this chapter, we discuss the feelings commonly experienced by families of cocaine users. We also discuss some of the ways in which people try to manage life with a cocaine-dependent relative. We explain how sincere attempts to help the cocaine user frequently backfire and recommend ways in which family members can help both themselves and the user.

Family Responses to the Cocaine User

Anger

Anger is probably the most common feeling experienced by relatives of cocaine users. They feel manipulated, unloved, and abused; they resent playing second fiddle to a drug. "Ruth" summarized the feelings of many spouses of cocaine users:

> I used to love my husband. He was a warm, kind, generous man. He loved me and he loved our children. But since he started using cocaine, he has turned into a monster. He screams at me and the children for no reason at all, and he constantly threatens us. He has stolen my jewelry and he went into my daughter's savings account and stole all of her babysitting earnings. The only sex he ever wants is with his coke whores, and because of him, I never answer the phone for fear of being harassed by a bill collector or threatened by a loan shark. I have no love for this man anymore, only hatred.

Guilt

One difficulty that some family members have in experiencing or expressing anger is their profound sense of guilt, which stems from their belief that they are somehow responsible for their relative's continuing drug use. Frequently parents, spouses, and children believe that if they had only acted properly their relative would never have become addicted. Certainly, most cocaine users are happy to accept this theory. They frequently blame their difficulties on their perceived mistreatment by others, rarely accepting the fact that their addiction is responsible for their misfortune. Many family members are only too eager to believe the cocaine user when he or she says that his or her fate is in their hands. By accepting this theory, they believe (mistakenly) that they have some ability to control this terrible illness that is ruining their family.

Fear

As cocaine dependence worsens, family members become increasingly afraid: afraid for their relative, afraid for themselves, and afraid for the family as a whole. As "Alexander," the father of one young cocaine user, said,

> I never knew from one night to the next what was going to happen. I stayed up till all hours of the night, waiting for her to come home, not sure whether I wanted her to or not. As long as she wasn't home, I knew that something terrible was happening to her, but at least I didn't have to see it. When she did get home, I knew that she wasn't out on the street doing God knows what, but then I would be physically afraid for my wife and myself, because she blamed all of her troubles on us. She went on rampages and threw plates all around the house, and I never knew if she would finally snap and try to kill us.

Shame

As an individual's cocaine dependence worsens, family members frequently become more and more despondent and hopeless. Their feelings about themselves may be characterized by self-blame, a sense of inadequacy, and at times self-loathing. They may believe that the cocaine user has disgraced the entire family, symbolizing their failure as parents, spouses, or children. Linda, a 14-year-old girl whose mother was dependent on cocaine, said,

> It got to the point where I couldn't bring other kids over to my house. My mother would sneak around, whispering about people out to get her, and there would always be some strange, sleazy-looking guy hanging around. She was nasty to me and all of my friends, and she used to call me names like "slut" in front of my friends for no reason at all. I'm sure that people must have looked down on me because of my mother, and the only way I knew how to handle it was to not let friends come over. It's hard to do, though, because after a while, people will stop inviting me over to their houses if I never ask them back. But I don't want to get the reputation as some creep or crazy person because of my mother.

The isolation that this young girl experienced is common in the families of drug users and can lead to a great sense of loneliness. As we shall see, this pattern of shame leading to isolation and loneliness is a particularly dangerous one, because it may lead the relative to believe that the only way to rescue his or her own life is by "rescuing" the cocaine user. As we shall see, not only is this an impossible task, but—paradoxically—it frequently allows the drug dependence to worsen.

How Families Try to Avoid the Pain of Cocaine Dependence

Denial

When faced with the painful feelings of anger, guilt, fear, and shame, family members frequently seek a way out. The fastest escape from these feelings is the same mechanism used by the cocaine-dependent person: denial. Denial in the family can take many forms. For example, relatives may join in with the user's denial by blaming his or her problems on other people, the user's job, the police, too much pressure—anything other than cocaine use. One frequent target of this misplaced blame is the family itself. This occurs partly because many relatives accept the role of scapegoat for the addicted person's difficulties.

Why would a family member accept blame for something that an impartial observer would say he or she did not cause? The following example illustrates this phenomenon and the reasons behind it: "Linda" was a 29-year-old attorney whose cocaine use was clearly causing her difficulties both at work and at home. She was alternately depressed and angry, she frequently missed deadlines at work, she alienated and lost clients, and she fought with her husband about virtually everything. Her husband, a passive and quiet man, rarely made demands on her because he knew it would create strife. He accepted her explanation that excessive job pressure had rendered her unable to cope with even minimal stress. He therefore bent over backward to lighten her load at home. When he realized that she was using much more cocaine than he had previously believed, he suggested that she cut down. This infuriated her, so he purposely did not bring up the subject again for several months, believing that "nagging" her would only increase her drug use. When he discovered that her cocaine use was escalating anyway, he discussed it with her again and suggested that she seek help. She refused to do so, and began to blame her drug use on her husband's "incessant harping." Although he initially accepted this explanation, he ultimately gained some perspective after she had entered treatment and stopped using cocaine. He described his reaction when she blamed him for her drug problem:

When she blamed me, it actually gave me a strange sense of hope. I thought, "If this is my fault in some way, then I have the power to make her stop using cocaine." How was that consoling? If I weren't influencing her, then all I could do was watch her throw her life and our marriage away. That prospect was a lot worse than feeling like I had some responsibility for her drug use.

Denial may also occur because relatives do not want to acknowledge that a loved one has a serious drug problem. Because so many people see addiction as an untreatable disease with terrible social stigma attached to it, acknowledgment of it in a family member may initially seem unbearable. Relatives therefore look for an alternative explanation for erratic behavior, difficulties at work, mood swings, paranoia, unexplained weight loss, disappearing money, and odd sleeping habits rather than face the fact that they have an addicted relative. Thus denial in the family is frequently a defense against fear: fear of helplessness against the disease and fear of the connotations and consequences of addiction.

Enabling

When the seriousness of an addiction makes denial impossible to maintain, a new pattern of behavior may appear in the family. Because of a strong sense of fear and guilt, relatives may begin to cover up for the patient's addiction, attempting to minimize the consequences that the addicted relative experiences as a result of the drug use. Family members may take over some of the responsibilities of addicted relatives, shield them from creditors, rescue them from drug-related legal difficulties, and perhaps go so far as to use drugs with them in an attempt to keep them "off the streets." This type of family behavior is generally called *enabling*, because shielding the addicted relative from the adverse consequences of drug use may actually support the addiction.

To understand this last statement, we need to explain why cocaine users generally seek treatment. They do not ordinarily stop using the drug merely because they feel they are using "too much." Cocaine is too powerful and too reinforcing to be given up without having compelling reasons for doing so. Therefore, it is frequently necessary for an individual to either have a meaningful loss or be threatened with such a loss before he or she will cease using the drug. If cocaine users believe they can continue to use the drug with impunity, they will be much less likely to stop. What are some examples of enabling behavior? Dr. Charles Nelson has listed six patterns that are frequently seen in the relatives of cocaine users:

1. *Avoiding and shielding.* This involves an attempt to prevent the cocaine user from experiencing the adverse consequences of drug use. Examples include hiding or throwing away cocaine and making up excuses to the user's friends and employer to cover up.
2. *Attempting to control.* This may include a variety of efforts such as screaming, making bargains or threats, leaving the house periodically, withholding sex, buying things for the user to divert his or her attention, or constantly staying with the user to control the amount of his or her drug use.
3. *Taking over responsibilities.* This typically involves taking over a variety of personal responsibilities for the cocaine user, such as paying bills, performing household tasks, waking the user in time for work, or covering debts.
4. *Rationalizing and accepting.* Relatives deny the severity of the drug use; some may even convince themselves that cocaine has made the user more communicative, more sexually attractive, or more creative.
5. *Cooperating and collaborating.* Relatives become directly involved with the drug use, helping the user to pay for, prepare, or use cocaine.
6. *Rescuing and subserving.* This consists of overprotectiveness to the point of making one's own needs secondary to those of the addicted relative. An example of this type of behavior would be cleaning up the cocaine user's vomit after a binge with cocaine and alcohol.

"Donna" unsuccessfully tried a variety of enabling behaviors to get her husband "Larry" to stop his cocaine use. At no time was she aware that her attempts to help him were backfiring. Rather, she felt that the failure of her efforts reflected her inadequacy as a wife. In her words,

> I first began to suspect that there was something wrong in our marriage when Larry started going out at night without me. We had always gone out separately once a week with our friends, and I had liked that arrangement. But when he started wanting to go out two

or three times a week without me, I suspected that he was seeing another woman. We had only been married three years, but I figured that something had to be missing in our marriage, and I naturally assumed that there was something wrong with me. Why else would a man go out that often without his wife? I never suspected at first that he was using cocaine. I knew that he used it every once in a while, and I had used it socially with him a few times. But it never seemed like a big deal.

I first began to suspect that he had a cocaine problem when we started having money problems. I would ask Larry why there seemed to be so little money left over from his paycheck, and he would just get mad at me and blame me for being a nag. I started getting more and more insecure and tried being nicer to him, figuring that maybe I had been kind of bitchy toward him. I started buying him surprise presents even though we were low on money. I tried to make all of his favorite foods, and I even tried doing different sexual things that I knew he wanted even though I wasn't really comfortable with them. [At this point, Donna was subserving herself to her husband. She was also not recognizing her anger at him because of her fear that she was losing him and because of her guilt that it was her fault.]

As time went on, it seemed like I couldn't do enough. No matter what I did, he kept going out, and he went out more and more often. When he came home, he would be irritable and would barely talk to me. Meanwhile, I found out that he wasn't paying any bills, although he had always been good about that in the past. We started getting letters from collection agencies and I started getting harassed by bill collectors on the phone. When I brought this up to him, he would just yell at me, so I started paying as many bills as I could out of my own paycheck, hoping that things would somehow straighten out. [Donna was now taking over responsibilities for her husband, still unaware of what was happening, but clearly afraid for herself and her marriage.]

One night, Larry didn't come home, and I got really upset. I was sure that he was out with another woman, and I didn't know if I could stand living with him under such circumstances. The next day when he came home, he denied being out with someone else, but admitted that he was using coke. Then he blamed the whole thing on me, saying that I wasn't enough fun, that I was too uptight sexually, and that I wouldn't use cocaine with him, so he had to do it with his friends. I figured that maybe I could help him to control the amount of cocaine he was using if I used some with him. That way, I could keep an eye on him and keep the problem from getting out of hand. [Donna was now attempting to control his use by co-operating and collaborating with him.] For a while, I thought things were getting better. Larry seemed a little calmer and happier than before, and I figured that at least he wasn't out with other women. [She was now rationalizing and accepting his use.]

It didn't take long for things to get really disastrous, though. His habit kept getting bigger and the trouble kept worsening. As he stayed home using his cocaine, we became social recluses. Friends would call us up to do things, and I would make up one excuse after another to try to avoid seeing them. [She was now avoiding and shielding.] I tried threats, blackmail, bribery, per-verted sex, using drugs with him, not using drugs with him, threat-ening to kill him, threatening to kill myself, leaving the house for a few days—everything I knew in order to get him to stop—but nothing helped. It was as if he didn't even notice that I was alive. Eventually, he started getting into trouble at work, and his boss was a lot more secure than I was. He just told Larry to get into treat-ment or give up his job. When it was put that way, Larry started treatment the next day, because he loved his job and because he knew that his boss meant business.

What is wrong with enabling? There is generally nothing wrong with the motivation behind the behavior or the diligence with which the effort is made. Family members of cocaine-addicted indi-viduals are desperate, and they work terribly hard to try to get their relatives to stop using cocaine. However, when they use the methods that Donna used, they are almost always doomed to fail. A term that has been used by some to describe relatives who use these enabling behaviors is *codependent*. This term implies that family members may also be made ill by the addictive process and that they themselves need help to recover from the devastating effects of this illness.

Deciding when to "help out" an addicted relative and when to let him or her fall can be an extremely complicated and painful task for relatives. These issues are illustrated in the following case example. Mr. and Mrs. "Smith" began to suspect that their son, "Bob," was in trouble when they noticed money missing from their wallets. They knew that he "fooled around" with drugs, but they did not confront him because they were afraid of what they might find if they delved too deeply. Eventually, Bob was arrested for dealing cocaine; his father hired the best criminal attorney available to defend him. Bob was acquitted, but two months later, he was arrested again on the same charges. He was bailed out of jail by his parents; they hired the same attorney, who was again able to obtain Bob's acquittal. Four days later, Bob was in an intensive care unit, recovering from a cocaine overdose.

Did Mr. and Mrs. Smith act wrongly by trying to keep their son out of jail? Would Bob have stopped cocaine sooner if he had not been bailed out of jail and had been forced to accept a public defender? No one can answer this. Bob's parents did what the vast majority of people would have done in the same situation. They tried to keep their son from suffering the possibly irreparable harm of incarceration, fervently hoping that he would use his arrests as a warning signal of what might happen to him. They hoped that he would change his behavior in order to avert a worse scenario at a later date.

Unfortunately, events that Mr. and Mrs. Smith interpreted as frightening portents were viewed by Bob as evidence of his charmed existence. When asked during treatment about his arrest, he said,

> I knew that nothing was going to happen to me. When I got off after the first bust, it became clear to me that nothing really bad was going to happen. Here I was, caught red-handed making a cocaine deal, and I walked away from it. I figured if I could beat that charge, I could beat anything.

The problem with enabling behavior is that it allows the addicted person to feel omnipotent; it reaffirms what we term the *pathological optimism* of cocaine users: feeling that they will land on their feet, no matter what happens to them. Because enabled cocaine users do not believe that future use will lead to adverse consequences, they are less likely to stop using the drug.

How Relatives Can Help

One of the harmful aspects of enabling behavior is the fact that shielding the cocaine user from the adverse consequences of his or her drug use may allow initially manageable problems to become uncontrollable. Thus, many addicted individuals who have been enabled do not seek treatment until they have suffered irreparable harm: serious physical damage, loss of a valued job, or jail. Meanwhile, their families have been hurt and embittered to an degree that is similarly difficult to repair.

Although some clinicians believe that cocaine users do not become motivated to stop their drug use until they "hit bottom" and lose everything, most people in the addictions treatment field believe that this scenario can be avoided through the process of *intervention*. Intervention involves confrontation of users by their family (or employer; see Chapter 7) for them to learn how their behavior has adversely affected their own welfare and their family members' lives. At an intervention meeting, family members and friends may gather together with the cocaine user and a professional—typically a physician, psychologist, or social worker experienced in such work. They then present the cocaine user with 1) clear, non-judgmental documentation of the results of his or her substance abuse; 2) treatment options that would be acceptable to the family; and 3) a clear statement of the family's response if he or she either refuses treatment or continues his or her substance use.

Interventions are emotionally charged, extremely difficult meetings in which the cocaine user often feels attacked and sometimes feels unloved. Family members may worsen the situation by seeing the intervention meeting as their chance to finally obtain revenge on the person who has made their lives so miserable. The presence of a skilled professional is important in such a meeting to ensure that the individual in question really has a substance abuse problem and to help the addicted person hear the genuine concern of his or her family, not just attacks. When all goes well, the evidence presented may prove overwhelming enough to convince the addicted relative that he or she has a problem that needs to be taken seriously. Ideally, he or she may decide to enter treatment immediately. It is thus important that no intervention take place unless there is an opportunity for immediate access to treatment, as the impact of the intervention can otherwise be quickly lost.

Another possible outcome of an intervention is that the addicted individual agrees to stop his or her substance abuse, but refuses to enter any or some of the treatments suggested. Thus, for example, the individual may agree to undergo psychotherapy, but will not attend a self-help group or a drug program. Alternatively, the individual may say that he or she will stop using drugs on his or her own, without the aid of any sort of treatment. The family should decide before the intervention how they will respond if this occurs, because a partial agreement of this nature is a common response. Family members must be ready to state what they will and will not tolerate and what is and is not negotiable. In some cases, the family may decide to not allow the individual back into the home until he or she has sought treatment.

A third possible result of an intervention is that the cocaine user will continue to deny the seriousness of his or her drug abuse and will thus refuse to stop using. Although such cases are initially discouraging, many of these families nevertheless benefit from the act of carrying out the intervention. This may represent the first time that family members have honestly and forthrightly attempted to face the reality of their relative's addiction. Because families of addicted individuals are frequently plagued by codes of silence, bickering, scapegoating, and mutual blaming, the opportunity for family members to speak openly about their feelings in a supportive environment can be extremely important. Another helpful aspect of the intervention is the fact that relatives are educated about the effects of substance abuse on the individual and the family. They may also be introduced to sources of ongoing support that are available to them in the community. These include Al-Anon, Nar-Anon, and Coke-Anon: organizations designed for the family members of individuals with alcohol and drug problems.

Perhaps the most important benefit of the process of intervention is the resolution by family members to stop enabling their relative's addiction. This may involve refusing to pay the addicted relative's bills, refusing to lie to protect his or her social or business reputation, or refusing to live in the same house with him or her. As one woman said to her husband in an intervention meeting,

> We are offering you one final chance to turn your life around. We have suffered too much as the result of your addiction. We love you and hope that you will get help so that we can live again as a family in peace. If you decide to get treatment, we will support you every step of the way. On the other hand, if you choose to continue using drugs, we have decided that we will no longer support your drug use in any way, because it hurts you and it hurts us. If you decide to return to drugs, then we'll focus on getting our own lives together.

Taking such a stand can initiate recovery for the family, and may eventually help the cocaine user to seek help.

Recovery for the Families of Cocaine Users

Although it may be quite dramatic, an intervention represents only the beginning of the long-term recovery process for the cocaine user and his or her family. Cessation of cocaine use does not remove the memories, distrust, and pain that occurred during periods of active drug abuse. Recovery also creates the need for adjustments in the family, because relatives have learned to adapt to life with an addict. For example, family members who endure chronic chaos and abuse may develop a sense of pride in their ability to tolerate disaster. They may thus paradoxically feel less "special" when their burden is taken away from them. Relatives may also become quite resentful when the addicted person starts to regain some self-esteem and begins to feel good about himself or herself soon after entering treatment. As the spouse of one cocaine user said, "How dare he feel so proud of himself after he has ruined my life for the last five years!" Some who have been hurt by their relatives want revenge, but they rarely find satisfaction in it.

For these and other reasons, support for family members of cocaine users is extremely important, both for them and for the recovery of the addicted relative. This may consist of psychotherapy, counseling, or Al-Anon, Nar-Anon, or Coke-Anon meetings. These last three groups support relatives of substance users by encouraging them to take care of themselves rather than trying to take care of their addicted relatives. These meetings, which can be attended by relatives or friends of active or recovering substance users, are guided by the same 12-step recovery program as Alcoholics Anonymous and Narcotics Anonymous. One of the most important guiding principles is the first step to recovery: "We admitted we were powerless over alcohol [drugs, cocaine]—that our lives had become unmanageable." Members of Al-Anon are encouraged to resist enabling by reminding themselves of the "three C's": they did not cause their relative's addiction, nor can they control or cure it. They are thus encouraged to "detach with love": to gain control over their own lives by realizing their inability to control the life of the addict.

Lasting recovery does not come easily. Family members must be prepared to deal with relapses on the part of the cocaine user and their own temptation to return to familiar but maladaptive coping mechanisms such as enabling. Relatives may try to "protect" the recovering individual from stress because of their fear that he or she will return to drugs if they become upset with him or her. Families who have argued constantly for years may not know how to interact when there is nothing to fight about. Some of these problems can be dealt with in ongoing family meetings, led by a professional who is experienced in family therapy. Families who have never communicated honestly and openly may need help and support to begin and continue this process.

The following case example illustrates one of the common pitfalls in the recovery process for families. In cases such as this, family therapy can help heal the wounds caused by chronic drug abuse: "Barbara," a 26-year-old woman with a history of cocaine dependence, had been drug free for one year. She was successful in her career and lived in her own apartment. She and her parents attended family therapy together because of the great difficulty they had experienced in talking to each other after her parents had learned of her cocaine use. At one meeting, Barbara's mother said, "I'm scared to put pressure on Barbara because I'm afraid she won't be able to handle it." This occurred shortly after Barbara had told her mother about a very painful problem she had endured with her boyfriend, an incident that she had handled with great aplomb and maturity. Barbara became quite upset and said, "Mom, you're doing now what you accused me of doing for years, which was not speaking my true feelings. You don't talk to me about painful stuff because you can't handle it." Her mother was encouraged to speak more honestly and openly to her daughter, and to worry less about Barbara's fragility. With time, she was able to do so, and was pleased to see that both she and Barbara could tolerate such an exchange.

Chapter 7

Cocaine in the Workplace

With the increased availability and decreased price of cocaine in the past decade, cocaine use has spread to many areas of society, including the workplace. Surveys reveal that, along with alcohol and marijuana, cocaine is one of the most common drugs of abuse among those who use drugs in a work setting. The large number of referrals of cocaine users to employee assistance programs (EAPs) and drug treatment centers tends to confirm this impression: a national survey of EAP caseloads found that 20% to 25% of their referrals were for cocaine addiction.

In general, the scope of drug and alcohol use in the workplace is quite extensive and disturbing, with estimates ranging from 10% to 25% of workers in the United States sometimes using drugs or alcohol on the job. The U.S. Department of Labor reported in 1989 that businesses that used drug testing found 10% of job applicants and employees testing positive for drugs. The social and economic cost to our society from drug use at work is enormous. Although highly speculative, several reports have estimated that the cost of alcohol and drug use in terms of lost productivity, job-related accidents, claims for health care benefits, and poor employee morale may be more than $50 billion per year.

Because cocaine may be used by individuals in a wide range of professions and job environments, this unfortunately includes occupations in which cocaine intoxication presents a danger not only to the user but to the general public as well. Specifically, occupations with long hours and high levels of tension, intermixed with boredom, provide fertile ground for the development of on-the-job cocaine use. As a result, air traffic controllers, pilots, workers in nuclear power plants, ambulance drivers, physicians, and nurses have all been noted to be at high risk for cocaine abuse.

Why Cocaine?

The reasons for cocaine's intrusion into the workplace relate both to social factors and to the properties of the drug itself. Despite increasing education about the dangers of cocaine use, the drug still carries a glamorous image for some people. Status-conscious adults who grew up in the drug culture of the 1960s and 1970s, and whose earlier experiences with marijuana, hallucinogens, and alcohol have prepared them for subsequent experimentation with other drugs, have been prey to the allure of cocaine. Indeed, within some peer groups, cocaine use is a socially sanctioned behavior, much the same way alcohol use is for other segments of our society.

Cocaine use in the workplace is facilitated by the fact that quantities sufficient to produce multiple episodes of intoxication can be transported in a small vial or aspirin bottle. In addition, the act of consuming the drug can be accomplished in seconds, with intoxication occurring almost instantaneously. Moreover, individuals who are "high" on cocaine frequently believe that despite being intoxicated, they are capable of "normal" functioning, both interpersonally and intellectually. Most important, they believe (sometimes correctly) that their intoxication is not apparent to those around them. In contrast, use of drugs like heroin, hallucinogens, or phencyclidine (PCP) is commonly known to render the user nonfunctional and thus their use easily detectable.

Another appealing property of cocaine is the fact that its use in low-to-moderate doses generally produces euphoria, increased alertness, and a sense of well-being. As a result, difficult tasks may seem easier, and boring repetitive tasks can be performed more rapidly. Jobs that require sustained attention can also be done more quickly, although often less carefully.

Hazards of Cocaine Use in the Workplace

Cocaine use, in either a social or occupational setting, is not without hazards, many of which have been described in previous chapters. In this chapter, we focus on the drug's effect on work performance and relationships with co-workers. As we discussed in Chapter 4, cocaine use can have detrimental effects on the body, especially the brain. As a result, cocaine use can affect cognitive functioning: one's ability to think and to learn and recall information. Cocaine users themselves report that cocaine can affect their cognitive abilities. When 500 callers to the 1-800-COCAINE hotline were surveyed, more than half reported impairment in memory and concentration as a result of cocaine use. A recent study at Yale University verified these subjective reports. Twenty heavy cocaine users received neuropsychological testing (specific tests of cognitive functioning) between 5 and 60 days after their last cocaine use. Half of those tested showed distinct deficits in attention and memory. Obviously, cognitive difficulties could seriously affect work performance, especially in individuals whose jobs demand alertness and focused attention.

In addition to cognitive impairment, other aspects of cocaine use can affect an individual's work performance. The following case illustrates some of these effects, as well as shows how the development of cocaine dependence can be both facilitated and interrupted by work-related factors: "Carl," a 30-year-old car salesperson, entered treatment because of a three-year history of cocaine abuse. He had reluctantly agreed to seek help at the insistence of his father, who owned the car dealership in which he worked. His father accompanied him to his first treatment session. Although Carl initially said he used cocaine only for "recreational" purposes on weekends, he grudgingly admitted that within the past three months, he had begun using the drug at work and that this had perhaps interfered with his performance. His father was more definite, characterizing the past several months as a financial and social disaster.

The youngest of three siblings, Carl described himself as a shy young man who had had aspirations to be a teacher. He was discouraged from pursuing a teaching career by his father and two older brothers, all of whom worked successfully in the family's automobile dealership. His inability to assert himself within the family was paralleled by awkwardness in social situations, particularly with women. Three years previously, he had been offered cocaine at a party and reluctantly agreed to try the drug so that others would not feel that he was a "wimp." He enjoyed the euphoria and sense of increased confidence he experienced after taking the drug. Later, he used cocaine again in similar circumstances on weekends.

As time passed, Carl's cocaine use increased in frequency from once or twice a month to every weekend. It was particularly heavy before, and during, social occasions. He felt that the drug made him more assertive and thus more comfortable with women. He also noted that while on cocaine, he was able to be more assertive with his father and brothers and felt less "pushed around" by them. These experiences reinforced his belief that cocaine had a useful therapeutic effect for him.

As Carl's weekend cocaine use increased, he noted that Mondays were difficult, in that he experienced low mood, fatigue, and difficulty concentrating on his work. Although he did not associate these difficulties with cocaine withdrawal, he began using a "line" or two on Monday mornings to "get going." He then noted that he was becoming more assertive and selling more cars. He was soon named "salesman of the month," thereby winning the respect of his father and brothers.

Over the next six months, Carl's cocaine use gradually increased in frequency to the point at which he was using the drug several times a day. His fellow workers began to note that in addition to being more assertive, he was also somewhat irritable and suspicious. His abrasiveness began to offend potential customers, some of whom complained to his father. His drug use on weekends also increased so that he was almost continuously intoxicated from Friday night until Monday morning. Moreover, although cocaine had previously enhanced his ability to socialize, he now preferred to use the drug while alone in his room, emerging only to replenish his supply or to meet with friends who were also cocaine users. A newly found girlfriend left him, telling his brothers that he was "acting weird" and that on several occasions he had been physically violent toward her as a result of cocaine-induced paranoia. At this point, his family confronted him about his drug use, which he minimized. Finally, at a stormy business meeting, he was confronted about his dwindling sales and poor attitude. He reluctantly agreed to seek help as an alternative to being fired.

This case illustrates some typical features in the development of cocaine dependence. Many individuals who experience uncertainty in interpersonal situations, who have difficulty "standing up" to their boss, or who feel chronically "put down" find that cocaine elevates mood, raises their self-esteem, and provides a false sense of security in interpersonal situations. Thus, in the beginning, cocaine use may actually help in overcoming real or imagined problems with initiative, assertiveness, or self-confidence. As a result, there is a tendency to turn to cocaine repeatedly in times of stress and to impart to the drug healing or restorative powers. Over time, however, the number of work-related or social situations that "require" pretreatment with cocaine increases to the point where the user feels unable to function properly without the drug.

As the cocaine user is gradually seduced, he or she may begin to lose sight of the drug's detrimental effects on work performance. The personality changes that accompany cocaine use (see Chapters 4 and 5) and the financial burden imposed by regular use also take their toll. In particular, long-term users may develop significant dependence on the drug. Such individuals, even if not intoxicated at work, may spend their work day preoccupied with obtaining cocaine or anticipating its use. As in the case of Carl, they may also begin to experience the rebound depression that often accompanies cocaine withdrawal. This in turn may lead them to use the drug in the morning before going to work.

As anticipated or actual drug use occupies more and more of the work day, there is a corresponding falloff in work performance as users experience drug effects, withdrawal symptoms, or apprehension about being caught. Despite these complications, users typically feel that they are functioning as well as, if not better than, they did before the onset of regular use. However, their supervisors frequently do not share this view. Thus it comes as a great surprise when they are passed over for promotion or fired outright as a result of sloppy work performance or deteriorating personal relationships with fellow employees and clients.

Carl's case also illustrates the potential power of an *intervention* (see Chapter 6) in the workplace, in which an employee is confronted about his or her drug use by a supervisor and is required to either enter treatment or lose his or her job. Carl, like many other cocaine users, was able to admit his problem only after being confronted in this manner.

Cocaine Use by Executives

Although drug abuse, per se, has traditionally been regarded as a problem for people in the lower socioeconomic classes, there is growing recognition that the problem is not confined to any social group. Indeed, data from EAPs and drug rehabilitation centers have shown that drug abuse by executives and professionals is a significant problem. Moreover, users include not only young middle managers, but corporate directors as well.

Why would an otherwise successful business executive be attracted by the lure of cocaine? The popularity of cocaine among some business executives stems from a variety of factors. These include the easy transportability of the drug, the fact that it can be self-administered within a matter of seconds in a locked office or bathroom, and the widespread misconception that cocaine intoxication does not interfere with intellectual functioning or decision making. In addition, for some executives, cocaine's ability to elevate mood and enhance their feelings of competence makes the drug appear to be a useful adjunct in their attempts to impress a coworker or a board of directors. Moreover, the hyperactivity and grandiosity that often accompany long-term cocaine use do little to contradict this self-perception. Unfortunately, supervisors, fellow employees, and competitors frequently see things otherwise.

Another factor that may contribute to cocaine use by executives is that a growing number of them are members of the "baby boom" generation of the post-World War II era. This population group, which is now entering its middle years, has had substantial experience with the use of other psychoactive drugs. In the 1960s, when the baby boomers were adolescents and young adults, recreational use of marijuana and hallucinogens may have been socially acceptable within their peer group. For many, getting a job, marrying, and having children have not altered this view. This is particularly true in the large urban areas of both coasts, where young and middle-aged professionals congregate around universities and high-technology industry. Here there exists a social milieu in which the willingness to experiment with certain drugs, like cocaine, may be socially acceptable. In contrast to opioids or sedatives, which render the user nonfunctional for at least an hour or two, cocaine is sometimes seen as a drug that enhances social relationships.

In many respects, the upwardly mobile young executive is an inviting target for cocaine use. Job pressures, long hours, frequent travel, and fierce competition take their toll, not only on the individual but on his or her major sources of emotional support: family and friends. In the business world, being a good spouse or parent are virtues that often go unrecognized and unrewarded. Although lip service is paid to the value of recreation, "quality time" with family members, and the need for rewarding nonbusiness relationships, the intense competitiveness of the business world often makes such activities seem frivolous. Sometimes, cocaine use is initiated as a substitute for meaningful family or marital relationships. Not surprisingly, some successful executives experience themselves as increasingly isolated, with job-related achievement being their only measure of self-worth. In this context, the availability of a drug that promises not only to enhance work performance, but also to make emotional support unnecessary, is a powerful attraction.

With the transition from occasional to habitual cocaine use, the focus of one's energies gradually turns away from concerns about work or family life and toward ensuring one's cocaine supply. In the workplace, there is a tendency toward increased sharing of information with other users about sources of supply. Joint purchases are made with co-workers to avoid low-level street dealers and the risk of being "ripped off," arrested, or blackmailed. As preoccupation with cocaine accelerates, work performance begins to suffer, although the cocaine user may be unaware that his or her judgment and abilities are not what they should be. When criticized by others, the user may be defensive, perhaps paranoid. Some individuals begin to feel that supervisors or co-workers are conspiring against them; sometimes they are right.

A business executive in trouble with cocaine frequently finds himself or herself with no one to turn to. After several years of drug involvement have complicated what may have already been a difficult marital relationship, the cocaine user's spouse may no longer be emotionally available. In other instances, the spouse may also be a drug or alcohol user, and may thus be unable to offer emotional support when needed. The executive may then attempt to use cocaine as a "bargaining chip" in exchange for friendship, emotional support, or sexual favors from co-workers. A common scenario is the middle-aged businessman who begins to supply cocaine to his secretary or someone else lower on the corporate ladder. This may be a way of enlisting allies in a real or imagined corporate struggle or an attempt to recapture lost youth in a relationship based on drugs and sex. Some business subordinates may find cocaine use intoxicating and exciting, whereas others are intimidated enough to go along with it despite their better judgment.

The Response of Business

In addition to the personal costs of cocaine use, business losses due to drug-related decreases in productivity and faulty decision making probably amount to billions of dollars annually. Further, cocaine dependence imposes a heavy personal financial burden. As a result, users with access to company funds may divert these for their own use through embezzlement, double billing, or acceptance of bribes or kickbacks. In addition, managers whose decisions can influence stock prices or the cost of a company's goods or services may become targets for personal or corporate blackmail when their drug-related impairment becomes known to drug dealers or business competitors. Moreover, in some work settings, the use of illicit drugs, including cocaine, represents a risk not only to the employee and his or her company, but to the general public as well. Examples include bus and taxi drivers, airline pilots, nurses, physicians, police, and other professions in which public safety is jeopardized by the presence of an intoxicated worker.

The high cost attached to drug abuse in the workplace has prompted the business community to respond in a variety of ways. In some cases, preemployment urine testing for drugs of abuse is used, although the usefulness and cost-effectiveness of this approach in determining suitability of job applicants are controversial. Moreover, if there is reason to suspect ongoing drug abuse, random urine screening may serve as both a deterrent and a method of detection. Indeed, some companies are beginning to require urine testing after a work-related accident, for absences for undocumented illness, or after a perceived decrement in work performance. Currently, approximately 90% of Fortune 500 companies use some sort of drug-testing program. Moreover, some such companies require that their vendors also test their employees.

In the absence of more subjective measures, however, reliance solely on the results of urine testing can be both clinically and legally hazardous. For example, individuals who have used marijuana consistently can produce urine specimens with detectable levels of tetrahydrocannabinol (THC)—marijuana's active ingredient—for more than a month after stopping the drug. In fact, positive tests for THC have been reported in individuals who have merely been in a room where marijuana was smoked. Another difficulty with urine screening programs is deciding how to deal with the presence of drugs that are part of a medically prescribed treatment regimen (e.g., codeine-containing cough preparations), but that may also be abused. Finally, it should be noted that urine and blood tests are not foolproof; both false-positive and false-negative results can occur. Thus all positive tests should be rechecked with a confirmatory test using a different analytic method, such as gas chromatography-mass spectrometry (GC-MS). Tests that remain positive require medical follow-up to determine whether further action, such as referral for treatment, is necessary.

The use of urine screening to detect drug-using employees is also complicated by civil rights issues. Not uncommonly, employees have refused to participate in blood or urine testing programs out of a sense of embarrassment or mistrust. Many are concerned about issues of confidentiality in the event of a positive test, and some have brought lawsuits against companies when the companies have taken punitive action on the basis of tests that the employees claimed were merely false-positive. In addition, there has been an ongoing debate as to whether widespread drug testing violates the constitutional rights of individuals. A United States Supreme Court ruling in 1989, however, upheld the constitutionality of drug testing of workers, even without individual suspicion of drug use.

The need for a practical approach to the problem of substance abuse in the workplace does not negate the need for firm limits on drug-using behavior. Many substance users, like Carl (see above), fail to appreciate the severity of their problem, and some fail to realize that a problem exists. As a result, they may need to be directly confronted not only by friends and family members, but by their employers as well. In this context, having to choose between getting help for a drug problem or losing one's job often provides the needed motivation to seek treatment. Under these circumstances, some companies require objective evidence that the employee is enrolled in a treatment program, whereas others require ongoing random urine screening for drugs of abuse. In such cases, urine samples may either be obtained through an outside treatment program or through the employee health clinic as a condition of continuing employment. Usually the company reserves the right to suspend or terminate any employee whose urinalysis indicates the continuation of illicit drug use. In some instances, the cycle of drug abuse needs to be interrupted by a brief period of hospitalization, a subject that we discuss further in Chapter 8.

The Concept of Employee Assistance

In the absence of a clear company policy that views substance abuse and other mental health problems as medical/psychiatric disorders (rather than moral infirmities), there is a tendency for supervisors either to look the other way when they suspect drug use or to harass suspected employees until they quit or transfer and become someone else's problem. In such an atmosphere, reporting may be precluded by a shortage of skilled workers, favoritism, or fear that one's own drug use will be exposed. Alternatively, peers may cover up for a drug-using co-worker so that the supervisor may be unaware of the problem. Eventually, however, absenteeism, poor work performance, and on-the-job intoxication present an overwhelming burden for co-workers and an unacceptable risk for the company.

In some organizations, the emphasis has shifted from dismissal of troubled employees to attempts at primary and secondary prevention of illness. Primary prevention efforts include wellness and stress management programs and other attempts to improve the general level of health and well-being of employees. Secondary prevention efforts are focused on the early identification and treatment of troubled employees. Some may already be involved in drug or alcohol abuse; others may be at increased risk for substance abuse as a result of associated mental health problems (e.g., depression) or a high level of life stress (e.g., recent separation or divorce). In an attempt to provide early identification and treatment for troubled employees with substance abuse or other mental health problems, a number of companies have developed, or contracted with, EAPs. These companies have decided that the cost of providing treatment for substance abuse or mental impairment in their employees is far less than the decreased productivity caused by these problems. The types of employee assistance available include telephone hotlines run by either paid counselors or volunteers, clinics that offer information and evaluation services to troubled employees and refer them for treatment outside the company, and in-house programs that provide comprehensive medical and psychological services. In a 1988 survey, the U.S. Department of Labor found that 30% of workers had access to an EAP, although workers in large businesses were more likely to have access to EAPs than those in small businesses.

Despite the increasing prevalence of EAPs, there have heretofore been few attempts to measure their effectiveness. Many barriers stand between the EAP and its use by employees. Many companies, including some with EAPs, view mental health problems—and particularly drug and alcohol problems—as a moral rather than a medical issue. Not surprisingly, some employees feel that if they seek help for emotional or drug-related problems, their confidentiality will be violated, their promotions will be jeopardized, and they may be fired. Although many EAPs rely on drug treatment programs that are independent of the company, confidentiality nevertheless remains an issue. Finally, in some instances, there is a lack of "marketing" of EAP services, so that employees are only dimly aware of the kinds of help available.

Despite their inherent difficulties, EAPs are generally quite helpful. By making evaluation and treatment services available to drug-dependent employees, EAPs also help to decrease the spread of substance abuse throughout their companies. Because drug-abusing employees are also frequently suppliers of illicit drugs, they are essentially "carriers" of the disease. The presence of rampant drug use within a company not only attracts other drug users as job applicants, but also sets up an atmosphere in which criminal activity may flourish. Prevention, early detection, and treatment efforts help to avert such situations.

When they work well, EAPs provide a valuable resource for drug-abusing employees and their supervisors. Ideally, they provide confidential evaluation and either on-site treatment or appropriate referral. They provide support and encouragement for employees undergoing active rehabilitation, and they serve as a link between the treatment program and the workplace. Thus the efficacy of treatment can be correlated with work performance. EAPs may, in addition, arrange for in-house meetings of Alcoholics Anonymous or Narcotics Anonymous for employees in varying stages of recovery from drug and alcohol dependence. EAP personnel may also establish close relationships with treatment programs in the community, thus allowing them not only to evaluate the results of treatment, but to identify the most appropriate treatment resources for their company's employees. Some EAPs also provide evaluation and referral for problems arising within the employee's family. These may include financial difficulties, marital infidelity, child abuse, and a host of other drug-related problems. Individual, couple, and family therapy may be indicated along with the use of outpatient support groups like Alcoholics Anonymous, Narcotics Anonymous, Al-Anon, Nar-Anon, and Alateen.

The EAP also provides a mechanism for monitoring both treatment compliance and posttreatment work performance. As a result, drug-abusing employees are less likely to "fall between the cracks." The existence of a monitoring component within the company also prevents supervisors from transferring problem employees to other parts of the company without revealing the nature of their problem. Such transfers are common practice in dealing with a disgruntled employee who denies drug use and who threatens to sue the company when he or she fails to get a desired promotion or when his or her employment is terminated. In short, a well-functioning EAP can provide a constructive alternative for addressing the problem of drug abuse in the workplace. This, in turn, fosters an atmosphere of concern and caring, rather than an adversarial relationship between the employee and the company.

In summary, the use of illicit drugs—particularly cocaine—is a significant problem, both for drug users and the companies that employ them. The response of management to this problem will do much to determine whether the work environment is one that fosters the initiation and maintenance of drug use or it is "therapeutic" in that it provides the structure and level of satisfaction necessary to facilitate the rehabilitation process. What is clear at present is that business cannot afford to ignore the problem of drug abuse in the workplace, and management needs to develop policies and procedures to address it. Approaches that consider the rights and best interests of employees, as well as those of the company, hold the most promise for success. Punitive approaches, which rely solely on detection and termination of employees, may merely drive the problem underground; in the long run, such programs are frequently not cost effective. The ubiquitous nature of substance abuse in our society makes consideration of these issues of paramount importance for the business community. Hopefully, they will continue to respond to the challenge with creative solutions.

Chapter 8

Treatment of
Cocaine Abuse

Although the cocaine epidemic is no longer a recent phenomenon, there is still relatively little known about the effectiveness of available treatments for cocaine abuse. In general, though, evidence suggests that cocaine addiction can be difficult to treat and that many people require intensive or repeated treatment to remain abstinent. Currently, most treatment for cocaine abuse takes place in general drug and alcohol treatment programs, which generally use techniques to treat cocaine users that are similar to those used for patients who are dependent on other substances. There are a few psychosocial and pharmacological treatment approaches, however, that have been developed or adapted specifically for cocaine abuse. We review these new treatment methods later in this chapter. Because research on cocaine abuse treatment is limited in many areas, much of what we describe as treatment for cocaine abuse is based on guiding principles that have been established for the treatment of a wide variety of addictive disorders.

One inherent difficulty in discussing the treatment of cocaine abuse is the fact that most people who use cocaine never seek treatment. Some people try the drug once or twice to satisfy their curiosity, and then never use it again. Others take the drug infrequently and experience no apparent adverse consequences. Still others experience temporary difficulties because of cocaine and decide to stop using the drug on their own. Thus a significant number of individuals stop using cocaine either because it does too little for them or because they are afraid that it may do too much to them.

We could learn a great deal about stopping cocaine use from those who quit the drug on their own: what motivated them, how they did it, and what helped. Unfortunately, however, because these individuals do not seek treatment, few of them have been formally studied. Further research on this population would be extremely valuable, therefore, because the patients seen in drug abuse treatment centers may represent only a fraction of the overall cocaine-using population.

What is the best treatment approach for those who cannot quit by themselves? Unfortunately, we cannot offer a single treatment prescription for all cocaine users. People who develop problems with cocaine are individuals, and they need treatment programs that are tailored to fit their own specific needs. Although certain people are able to stop using cocaine on their own, some require intensive treatment, such as inpatient treatment or partial hospitalization; others can be successfully treated as outpatients. In this chapter, we 1) discuss how and why cocaine users enter treatment, 2) describe the various types of treatment methods that are available, and 3) review some of the general principles involved in helping people to stop using cocaine.

Getting the Cocaine User Into Treatment

The first requirement of a successful cocaine abuse treatment program is that the patient enters treatment. Unfortunately, this may also be the most difficult aspect of treatment. As we discussed in Chapter 5 ("Cocaine Dependence"), addicted cocaine users frequently deny or minimize the extent to which their drug use is adversely affecting their lives. Thus they may not seek treatment until some event begins to break down that denial. Cocaine users do not ordinarily seek help merely because they feel they are using too much cocaine. Rather, they usually come to professional attention only after their cocaine use is undeniably creating a problem in some other aspect of their lives. Typically, cocaine use causes problems in one of the following areas, any of which may lead the user to seek treatment:

1. *Medical:* Because cocaine users are able to deny the importance of such "minor" difficulties as a perforated nasal septum, it may take a major, life-threatening medical problem, such as a grand mal seizure (convulsion), to alert them to the seriousness of the problem.

2. *Vocational:* Absenteeism, tardiness, and erratic job performance are common consequences of cocaine abuse. As employers learn more about substance abuse, they are more likely to recognize these patterns of behavior as potential symptoms of cocaine abuse. They may respond by making continued employment contingent on successful completion of a drug treatment program.

3. *Financial:* Cocaine use can be expensive, especially for those with serious addictions who use cocaine frequently. Unless one is extremely wealthy or willing to undertake illegal activity, it is very difficult to maintain such a habit. Unfortunately, some people do not enter treatment until they have fallen heavily into debt. For those who fund their addictions with criminal activity, legal problems may lead them to seek treatment.

4. *Legal:* For users who are not rich, the three major methods of maintaining a substantial cocaine habit are stealing, dealing, and prostitution. Thus many people enter treatment via the criminal justice system. One might instinctively think that such individuals would be unmotivated for treatment and have a relatively poor prognosis. However, this is not always the case as we will discuss below.

5. *Interpersonal:* As we discussed in Chapter 6, cocaine abuse can cause great damage to the family. Sometimes, the only leverage that a spouse can exercise in dealing with an addicted partner is the threat of separation. Sometimes, such a threat will lead a cocaine user into treatment. More often, however, the addicted spouse finds the threat unbelievable. If the ultimatum is being made for the first time, the user is likely to call the spouse's bluff. When threats have been made previously but not carried

out, the addicted spouse has "proof" in his or her own mind that there is no need to worry.

6. *Psychological:* Some people seek treatment because they are frightened by what cocaine is doing to them. They are worried by the direct drug effects (depression, hallucinations, paranoia, and delusions), and they are frightened by the erosion of their own values. For example, one patient came to our unit because he had overextended himself financially, and he was becoming increasingly tempted to sell his mother's jewelry to finance his habit. Fortunately, his level of denial and rationalization was not high enough to allow him to carry this out, and he sought treatment before he actually completed this act.

Sometimes friends, family members, employers, physicians, or others who are close to an addicted user do not wait for him or her to "hit bottom." Rather, they perform an intervention, the purpose of which is to help the user face the consequences of his or her own use. (Interventions are described in more detail in Chapters 6 and 7.) If this is unsuccessful, it may be helpful to create some adverse consequences in a controlled setting before the cocaine user loses so much that recovery becomes even more difficult. This process is sometimes referred to as "raising the bottom."

Unfortunately, just because an addicted individual enters treatment does not mean that he or she is a willing participant. Many of the aforementioned avenues into treatment are at least partially coercive; a major goal of treatment, therefore, is to instill some motivation into the patient. Even in our treatment center, in which we require the patient to call the hospital himself or herself to request admission, most patients coming into our unit would initially like nothing better than to get high. This is more easily understood when one realizes that most active, addicted cocaine users want to stop and most abstinent addicted users want to get high. What separates the two groups is the relative strengths of these conflicting emotions and, more important, the behavioral result of this inner battle. Thus many of our successful patients are discharged from the hospital with the desire to get high, but with the ability not to act on this wish.

Treatment Methods for Cocaine Users

Outpatient Treatment

The first major question one must answer in considering various treatment methods for a cocaine user is whether the drug problem can be managed on an outpatient basis or the patient will need to be hospitalized. Obviously, outpatient treatment is preferable to hospitalization whenever feasible, because it requires the expenditure of considerably less time and money and minimizes overall life disruption. On the other hand, inpatient treatment has the advantage of being far more intensive, and it removes the addicted patient from what is often a harmful life-style and from ready access to additional cocaine. In assessing an individual's capacity to successfully engage in outpatient treatment, we carefully examine his or her level of denial, commitment to treatment, and social supports, as well as the presence of coexisting medical or psychiatric problems that might make outpatient treatment less feasible.

In our experience, outpatient treatment has the best chance of success for patients who clearly recognize the destructive impact of cocaine on their lives and who enter treatment with a sincere desire to do whatever is necessary to stop using the drug. We initially attempt outpatient treatment with such patients, with the understanding that continued drug use may indicate the need for more intensive treatment.

How frequently should outpatient treatment be conducted? The results of one recent study suggested that once-a-week outpatient therapy may be insufficient to treat this patient population. Dr. Sung-Yeon Kang and co-workers in New York studied more than 100 cocaine-dependent patients in once-weekly psychosocial treatment; the patients engaged in either family therapy, individual supportive therapy, or group therapy. These researchers studied outcome 6 to 12 months after initiation of treatment and found that only 19% of the patients were not using cocaine at follow-up. On an optimistic, note, however, those who were abstinent from cocaine demonstrated significant improvement in many aspects of their functioning. This study concluded that unless an individual is highly motivated to stop using cocaine, more intensive (i.e., more than once a week) outpatient or inpatient treatment is generally necessary.

Within the broad category of "outpatient treatment" are numerous specific treatment methods that have been used with varying degrees of success with cocaine users and other drug-dependent individuals. In the following section, we discuss some of the most widely used techniques for treating cocaine users.

Individual psychotherapy. In individual psychotherapy, a patient and a psychotherapist (usually a psychiatrist, psychologist, or social worker) discuss a wide variety of personal problems, including the patient's drug use, difficulties with interpersonal relationships, and inner conflicts. Psychotherapy may focus on current life issues or may examine in depth the contribution of childhood experiences to current psychological difficulties. In general, psychotherapy with an active or newly abstinent cocaine user is likely to focus primarily on his or her current difficulties, at least at first. When stable abstinence has brought these crises under control, further exploration of the origins of the patient's problems can proceed more smoothly.

"Paul," a 31-year-old accountant, entered psychotherapy after his wife told him to either seek treatment for his cocaine use or leave the house. He had been treating his wife and son cruelly, was neglecting responsibilities at work, and had experienced numerous bouts of depression. The major focus of his first two months of psychotherapy was stopping his cocaine use. His therapist encouraged Paul to attend Narcotics Anonymous (NA) meetings, and they discussed the feelings, events, and places that stimulated his desire for cocaine. Paul's therapist also taught him techniques that could help him avoid drug use even when his craving for cocaine was high. As Paul's preoccupation with cocaine diminished with a lengthening period of abstinence, the focus of his psychotherapy began to shift toward the initial precipitants for his drug use: anxiety about becoming a father (he began heavy cocaine use during his wife's pregnancy) and his own unresolved relationship with his abusive alcoholic father. As he began to learn more about these issues, he gained a greater sense of mastery over his emotions, and his desire to escape from uncomfortable feelings decreased.

Relapse prevention therapy. Researchers at Yale University have found that individual psychotherapy seems to be effective in helping some cocaine-dependent individuals achieve abstinence. However, they found that a specific form of psychotherapy known as *relapse prevention therapy* may be more effective in leading to abstinence than more traditional forms of psychotherapy that use a supportive, "interpersonal" approach as described above. Relapse prevention treatment appears to be particularly useful for individuals with severe cocaine problems.

Initially used in treating alcoholic patients, relapse prevention treatment has been found to be useful in many different settings. The focus of relapse prevention is on developing "common sense" strategies to avoid situations and settings in which relapse to cocaine use would be likely. Initial interventions address the ambivalence most cocaine users have about stopping by helping them to see the negative consequences of their cocaine use. Then strategies are taught to help patients deal with their cocaine craving and to help them avoid situations in which they might develop urges to use cocaine. Finally, relapse prevention focuses on life-style changes that are necessary for the maintenance of cocaine abstinence.

"Sara," a 23-year old woman, sought outpatient treatment for cocaine addiction after she had been fired from two jobs in the course of 6 months because of frequent absences from work. She was assigned to a therapist who primarily used relapse prevention techniques. Initially, Sara reported that she was not sure that she had a "serious" cocaine problem and that she wanted treatment just to help her cut back on her cocaine use. Sara's therapist asked her to divide an index card in half, and on one side to list all the possible benefits of continued cocaine use and on the other side to write down all the possible reasons to stop cocaine use. Sara was amazed to see the length of the list of reasons to stop: she wrote down "I don't want to lose another job," "I would have more money," "My parents would stop yelling at me to stop using." She also realized that many of the possible benefits to continuing cocaine use actually had negative consequences. For example she had written, "I feel so good about myself when I'm high" but then realized that she had also written in her list of reasons to stop, "Sometimes when I'm really high I get very paranoid and feel really scared," and "I feel lousy the day after I've used a lot of coke." Sara's therapist instructed her to keep this index card in her purse and to look at it whenever she thought about using cocaine.

After three weeks of treatment, Sara decided that she wanted to stop using cocaine completely because too many negative consequences would ensue if she continued to use. Her therapist began to help her identify situations and places that she would have the opportunity or the desire to use cocaine. These included being with a particular group of friends who used cocaine and being near the house where she used to spend time with these friends using cocaine. Sara developed strategies to avoid driving close to this house; she also decided to spend her free time with another group of friends who did not use cocaine or other drugs. In addition, she realized that anytime she had more than $20 in her purse, she thought about using it to buy cocaine. She therefore decided to let her parents manage her money, and she asked them to give her only $15 at a time. Further, Sara's therapist discouraged her from trying to "test" her ability to remain abstinent, for example, by driving past the house where she used to use cocaine just to see if she was able to do it.

During this stage of treatment, Sara used cocaine on two occasions. She reported this use to her therapist, who helped her to look carefully at the chain of events that had led her to use. On one occasion, Sara reported that she had gone to a wedding at which alcohol was served. She had felt out of place not drinking, and she had told herself, "My problem's not really with alcohol, its with cocaine," so she had allowed herself to drink a few glasses of champagne. A short time later, she encountered one of her old cocaine-using friends who offered her cocaine. Sara reported that she "didn't think twice," but went ahead and used the cocaine. In discussing this with her therapist, Sara became very aware that she had to avoid drinking alcohol because it impaired her judgment and had led her to think she could use cocaine again.

After three months of therapy, Sara's treatment became more focused on the need to examine her life-style. Sara realized that without cocaine, she felt bored much of the time. She also felt that her circle of friends who did not use drugs was too small and did not provide her with enough fun. She was encouraged by her therapist to develop other interests and to engage in activities she found enjoyable. Sara remembered that during college she had loved to swim, and she decided to start swimming again. In addition, her therapist encouraged her to become more active in a Cocaine Anonymous (CA) group at which Sara had met several people whom she enjoyed. After six months of treatment, Sara was doing well and had not used cocaine for more than four months.

Behavioral therapy. A variety of behavioral strategies, some based on classical (Pavlovian) conditioning models and others based on operant conditioning, have been developed to help cocaine-dependent patients remain abstinent. *Cocaine cue extinction,* a treatment strategy developed by Dr. Anna Rose Childress and her colleagues at the University of Pennsylvania, focuses on diminishing addicted patients' classically conditioned responses to cocaine-related stimuli. When abstinent cocaine users are presented with stimuli previously associated with cocaine use, they typically report cocaine craving. These stimuli can include drug paraphernalia, drug-buying locations, or former drug-using friends. As a result, they are particularly vulnerable to relapse in these situations, even if they feel motivated to remain abstinent. Cocaine cue extinction involves systematically exposing patients to drug-related stimuli in a safe, controlled environment. By repeatedly exposing addicts to these stimuli in the absence of cocaine use, the strength of the association between the drug-related cues and actual use of cocaine should decrease over time.

Behavioral treatment based on an operant conditioning model has also shown some promise; preliminary research suggests that treatment that includes incentives to remain abstinent may be effective for some cocaine users. For example, researchers at the University of Vermont, led by Dr. Stephen Higgins, offered material incentives (vouchers to purchase material items) to addicted cocaine users who produced negative urine tests. They found that individuals receiving this form of behavioral treatment were better able to achieve abstinence than those offered counseling alone. Similarly, presenting an addicted patient with a negative consequence for ongoing use, a treatment modality known as *contingency contracting*, may also help him or her remain abstinent. Patients in this form of treatment who do not already have a clear negative consequence of further cocaine use help to design such a contingency themselves. Thus a patient might write a letter to his or her employer, detailing his or her history of drug use at work. This letter is then held by the therapist, who only mails it to the employer if the patient returns to drug use, as evidenced by positive urine screens.

Group psychotherapy. In group psychotherapy, 6 to 12 group members meet with one or two professional leaders to discuss both individual problems and relationships among themselves. Groups for drug-dependent patients usually offer peer support for remaining abstinent, advice on issues such as marital and vocational problems, and confrontation when group members perceive that someone is at risk to relapse. One advantage of the group approach is the fact that drug-dependent patients are adept at recognizing subtle signs of denial and self-deceit in each other, because they are so familiar with these behaviors themselves. One potential drawback of group therapy is the fact that some very passive or shy patients who find it difficult to talk in groups may not deal adequately with their own personal problems in this setting. Although the efficacy of group therapy for cocaine users has not been widely studied, preliminary results from a Harvard Medical School study suggest that group therapy helps keep patients in treatment and may offer substantial benefits.

"Steve," a 22-year old student, was referred for drug-oriented group psychotherapy because of a history of cocaine abuse and manipulative behavior. Because he was one of the youngest members of the group, he initially tried to impress other members by recounting "war stories" of his drug use; he reveled in describing his narrow escapes from arrest and serious injury. Other members of the group recognized his high level of anxiety and denial; they therefore offered him a useful combination of support and confrontation. As the group progressed, Steve attempted to exploit other group members, as he had done previously in other relationships. When the group members reacted negatively to this, he began to appreciate the adverse consequences of his manipulativeness. He subsequently made an effort to deal with others more honestly and genuinely.

Couples or family therapy. This treatment modality is particularly helpful in families for whom drug use has replaced or precluded other forms of communication. In some families, anger and resentment over one person's substance abuse can severely compromise the ability of family members to talk to one another about anything. In family or couples therapy, various members of a family meet with a professional to discuss the impact of the drug use on family members, to examine how family stresses are sometimes expressed by one person's drug use, and to help ease the difficulties that the drug user and the family both experience during recovery. (Further discussion of family therapy can be found in Chapter 6.)

Medication. The use of medications in the treatment of cocaine abuse has been the subject of intense interest. As scientists have learned more about the neurophysiological changes resulting from chronic cocaine abuse, there has been an increasing effort to discover how specific medications may help to correct these alterations. Although many different medications have been tried, the results have not yet been as encouraging as many had originally hoped. In certain situations, however, such as when another psychiatric disorder exists in addition to cocaine abuse, medication treatment can be very helpful.

Our own research has identified a significant subgroup of chronic cocaine users who concurrently have mood disorders: recurrent episodes of depression, or mood swings varying from highs to lows (bipolar disorder, formerly called *manic-depressive illness*). These studies, whose findings were replicated by other researchers, suggest that medications that are typically used to treat mood disorders may be helpful in this subgroup of cocaine users. Cocaine-dependent patients with depression can be effectively treated with

151

antidepressants such as desipramine or imipramine. Similarly, those with bipolar disorder or severe mood swings can be treated with lithium carbonate, which is typically prescribed in such disorders (although the effectiveness of lithium in reducing cocaine use in patients with bipolar disorder has been suboptimal). A psychiatric evaluation can therefore be extremely useful in helping to determine whether another potentially treatable disorder may be making a cocaine abuse problem worse.

The following case example illustrates the potential utility of medication treatment with certain cocaine-dependent patients: "Ann," a 27-year old laboratory technician, was hospitalized because of a three-year history of cocaine abuse. She stated that she had initially used cocaine at a party with a group of friends and had experienced a dramatic change in her mood. She said, "I never knew that I had been depressed until after I used cocaine. Then I finally knew what it was like to feel good." Unfortunately, the feelings of well-being caused by cocaine were short-lived, and she experienced steadily worsening mood swings as well as vocational, marital, and financial difficulties as a result of her cocaine abuse. She entered treatment on the advice of her employer.

Ann was extremely depressed at her admission to the hospital and experienced some suicidal thoughts. Unlike most patients, however, Ann's depression did not improve at all during the course of her hospitalization. Although she participated in individual psychotherapy, numerous groups, and NA meetings, she felt that she was "just going through the motions. I felt miserable and didn't really care if I got better." She complained of a poor appetite and weight loss while in the hospital, and she frequently awoke during the middle of the night and early in the morning. Because the latter symptoms are typically seen in non-drug users with mood disorders, and because we observed so little improvement in Ann's mood after two weeks of hospitalization, we treated her with the antidepressant drug desipramine at a dose of 150 milligrams a day. Within approximately two weeks, her mood gradually improved, she became much more hopeful, her sleeping and eating habits normalized, and her craving for cocaine diminished. She continued in individual psychotherapy and in NA and was able to use treatment much more to her advantage. She said, "My heart was in it now. I wanted to get better and I felt that I could."

In addition to the subgroup of cocaine users with concurrent mood disorders, some cocaine addicts have attention-deficit hyperactivity disorder (ADHD), adult residual type (see Chapter 4 for more details). ADHD is first present in childhood when an individual can be hyperactive, impulsive, and have trouble concentrating. Symptoms of this disorder sometimes persist into adulthood and cause ongoing difficulties with impulsiveness and concentration. We have found that some cocaine users with ADHD may be better able to abstain from cocaine when symptoms of their ADHD are treated with appropriate medications. These medications include pemoline (Cylert), methylphenidate (Ritalin), and tricyclic antidepressants, such as desipramine or imipramine. Although useful in treating ADHD, stimulant drugs must, of course, always be used extremely cautiously in cocaine users because they may stimulate cocaine craving.

For cocaine-dependent patients who do not have a concurrent psychiatric disorder, medication treatments remain promising. However, none of the approximately two dozen medications that have been used to treat cocaine dependence has proven to be universally effective. Pharmacological strategies have focused on trying to reverse the neurochemical changes in the brain that are thought to result from chronic cocaine use (see Chapter 4). In large part, medications that reverse derangements in dopamine activity have been used. The most effective medications in this regard have generally been tricyclic antidepressants, such as desipramine. Although these drugs are primarily used for treating symptoms of depression, research studies have suggested that these medications can be effective in some cocaine-dependent patients without significant depression, because of their effect on dopaminergic activity in the brain. For example, Dr. Frank Gawin and his co-workers reported in one study that desipramine decreased cocaine craving and facilitated the initiation of abstinence in cocaine-dependent patients. Unfortunately, the usefulness of desipramine is limited by the long period of time it takes before this medication is effective—typically two to three weeks after initiating treatment. This is a critical time during which many cocaine users relapse or drop out of treatment. Moreover, more recent studies have been less sanguine about the utility of this agent.

Other drugs that theoretically can reverse cocaine's effect on the dopamine system include L-tyrosine (the amino acid precursor of dopamine), bromocriptine, and amantadine (two drugs that have dopamine-like activity in the brain). When subjected to rigorous study, L-tyrosine has not been found to be beneficial in reducing cocaine craving or in helping addicted patients achieve abstinence, whereas research on bromocriptine and amantadine has generated mixed results. Other medications that affect the dopamine system, such as flupentixol and pergolide, show some promise in helping cocaine-dependent patients but are still in the early stages of study. Despite promising early reports regarding carbamazepine (Tegretol), an anticonvulsant drug, more rigorous study of this medication has not confirmed its beneficial effects in cocaine users. Finally, a drug that acts on the brain's opiate system, buprenorphine, may be effective in cocaine-dependent patients who also use heroin in a particularly dangerous combination known as a "speedball." Results from early studies have indicated that buprenorphine may reduce both heroin and cocaine use in this population, as well as reducing needle-sharing—a major risk factor for human immunodeficiency virus (HIV) infection. This drug, too, will need to be studied more extensively, however.

Acupuncture. Several preliminary studies have indicated that acupuncture may be helpful in reducing cocaine craving, particularly during the early phases of abstinence. Although we are still awaiting results from well-controlled, large-scale trials on this treatment method, it is possible that acupuncture may play a role in the treatment of patients with cocaine dependence.

Self-help groups. Alcoholics Anonymous (AA) and similar organizations, such as Narcotics Anonymous (NA) and Cocaine Anonymous (CA), are self-help groups whose aim is to help substance users achieve lasting sobriety. These worldwide organizations meet regularly so that members can share their recovery experiences and support each other in the struggle to avoid relapse. These programs support complete abstinence from all drugs, including alcohol. Unlike the help offered by many professionals and social agencies, these groups are almost continuously available. Experienced group members (sponsors) help to support newer members during periods in which the risk of relapse is high. During the group meetings themselves, members hear others' stories of recovery and often find their first rays of hope in one of these meetings. The only requirement for membership is the honest desire to become drug and alcohol free. There are no fees or dues. More recently, self-help groups that offer an alternative to the 12-step model of recovery espoused by AA have gained popularity. The most popular of these groups, which eschew the emphasis on spirituality and a "higher power," is Rational Recovery. Women for Sobriety is a self-help group for women who believe that their needs are not sufficiently addressed in what they see as the more traditional male-dominated AA.

The following case example illustrates one way in which self-help groups can be an important part of the treatment of cocaine dependence: "Cathy," a 30-year-old writer, was referred to NA by her family physician after she had told him about her steadily increasing cocaine habit. Cathy's reaction to her initial meeting was quite negative:

> I entered a smoke-filled room and saw a bunch of tough-looking guys and sleazy-looking women, and I was convinced that none of these people had anything in common with me. Looking back on it, I know that I purposely sought out people who were different from me in order to give myself an excuse to not get involved and not give up cocaine.
>
> At that first meeting, though, I managed to meet one woman who had a lot on the ball and was very helpful. She encouraged me to come back to NA again and see if I liked it any better. I was pretty resistant, but I knew that my cocaine habit was pretty bad, so I decided to give it one more try. The second meeting seemed a little less dreary than the first. When I heard the speaker, I heard a lot of things that reminded me of myself, and my ears picked up a little bit when she started to talk about her recovery. I listened in on other people's conversations, and when I started to hear recovery

stories, I began to think, "If these people can get straight, I can." I went again, and some faces started to look familiar. People started getting more friendly, and I realized that there was a lot of warmth in NA, and people really care about each other. There is this mentality that we're all in this boat together and that, by helping out each other, we help ourselves.

I struggled hard with the first step of NA, which involved admitting that I was powerless over cocaine and other drugs and that my life had become unmanageable because of my addiction. When I finally accepted this step, though, I started to get better. I got myself a sponsor and I call her regularly. I have a list of phone numbers of other NA members, and I keep in regular contact with a group of people, just so that I don't drift into trouble without my knowing it. I've made some good friends in NA, and I've had to give up my old drinking and drugging companions. I honestly believe that going to that first meeting saved my life.

Outpatient drug programs. These programs, which may be affiliated with inpatient facilities, usually offer individual or group therapy, family counseling, and urine screening. Outpatient drug programs are frequently staffed by recovering drug-addicted or alcoholic workers. Some outpatient cocaine programs have frequent group meetings (two to four times per week), require that their members attend a self-help group such as NA regularly, and ask for urine screens one to three times per week. The intensity of these programs is designed to combat the powerful drug craving that many people experience when initially trying to stop cocaine. These programs are also important for individuals who have been recently discharged from inpatient treatment to help them maintain abstinence.

Partial hospitalization. In recent years, many treatment centers have offered an intermediate level of care between inpatient and outpatient treatment. In these "partial hospital" programs (sometimes called *day treatment* or *evening treatment*), patients receive intensive outpatient treatment—commonly for six hours a day, five days a week. In most of these programs, patients sleep at home, but some partial hospital programs are affiliated with a residential treatment center where patients can go at night. The major advantage of partial hospital treatment, other than its reduced cost, is also a potential disadvantage; patients may be exposed to drug-related stimuli upon leaving and are thus tested on what they are learning in treatment. For many such patients, this motivates them to work harder in treatment. For some, early exposure results in relapse and dropout from treatment.

Inpatient Treatment

Hospitalization. For some individuals with severe cocaine problems, a hospital may offer the safest place for treatment to begin. Hospitalization is usually indicated when less intensive treatment has failed or when the patient's life circumstances make outpatient treatment either too risky or impossible. The following is a partial list of situations that would make us likely to recommend treatment in an inpatient facility. Hospitalization is usually recommended if cocaine users

1. Are actively threatening self-harm.
2. Are actively threatening to harm someone else.
3. Are taking such poor care of themselves that they represent a significant threat to accidentally harm themselves. This might include individuals who have recently begun to use drugs intravenously or who expose themselves to great physical danger in obtaining drugs.
4. Are dangerous to others and themselves because of their recklessness and poor judgment, such as individuals who regularly drive while intoxicated.
5. Have a poor system of social supports, such as individuals who live with other active substance users.
6. Have severe medical or psychiatric complications in addition to cocaine abuse.
7. Are dependent on alcohol or drugs other than cocaine and need medical detoxification.
8. Have failed in less intensive treatment.

Hospital treatment, which usually takes place on a specialized substance abuse unit, offers several advantages over outpatient treatment. First, the hospital environment offers a safe refuge from cocaine at a time when addicted patients are least capable of resisting the drug on their own. The decreased availability of cocaine reduces drug craving (see Chapter 5) and offers patients enough time to learn that they can make a choice about their drug use. Another advantage of hospitalization is the fact that the patients immediately become part of a supportive peer group of other addicted individuals who are similarly attempting to stop their drug use. Placement in a new, supportive environment offers them hope that they can overcome some of the loneliness and isolation that are so common among chronic drug users.

Family involvement is often a critical aspect of hospital treatment, as it is in outpatient or partial hospital treatment. Relatives and friends of cocaine users are frequently angry, depressed, and desperately frustrated. They, too, need a great deal of support and education about the addictive process, its effects on family members, and ways in which they can rebuild their own lives (see Chapter 6 for further discussion about the effect of cocaine addiction on the family).

In addition to repairing strained relationships with loved ones, another task of hospitalization is the assessment of the patient's vocational or school situation (see Chapter 7). Because so many cocaine users eventually experience difficulty at work because of their drug use, vocational counseling is an important part of a drug rehabilitation program. Involvement of the employer in this process is sometimes quite helpful in improving work attendance as well as performance.

One important benefit of inpatient treatment is the fact that patients can undergo extensive medical, neurological, and psychiatric evaluation while they are drug free. This is important in assessing and treating the common complaints of depression, anxiety, and insomnia, which are very difficult to evaluate in active cocaine users. It is initially virtually impossible to determine whether these symptoms are resulting from chronic cocaine use, from the withdrawal or "crash" that commonly follows the cessation of cocaine use, or from the numerous adverse events (e.g., loss of job, family, and finances) that so frequently occur in the lives of cocaine users.

Alternatively, these symptoms may have preceded the substance abuse and led to a misguided attempt at "self-medication" with cocaine or other drugs. In a drug-free hospital environment, we can begin to differentiate between the causes and effects of cocaine abuse and thus design a specific, individualized treatment program for each patient.

A final, critical advantage of inpatient care or partial hospitalizations is their intensity: the doctors, nurses, social workers, and counselors working in an inpatient program have the opportunity to interact with patients 24 hours a day and can therefore observe patients' reactions to frustration, sadness, anxiety, anger, and happiness. Very often, subtle stresses that cause drug urges in cocaine users may not be readily observable in once- or twice-weekly psychotherapy. However, patients who experience the desire to use cocaine while in the hospital can talk about this feeling immediately. They may thus begin to understand more fully the precipitants for their cocaine use and alternatives to giving in to their drug urges.

The following case example illustrates some of these points: "George," a 36-year-old contractor, admitted himself to the hospital after becoming suicidal when his wife threatened to divorce him if he did not stop his cocaine use. George had used a variety of drugs since adolescence, with cocaine predominating during the past five years. He had financed his habit through heavy drug dealing; a threat to his family as the result of a recent transaction had led his wife to present him with an ultimatum.

When George first entered treatment, he was highly unmotivated and said that the goal of complete abstinence was unrealistic:

> I thought the staff were fools to think that we were supposed to stop using everything. I was looking to get my cocaine use under some control, and I was willing to consider stopping cocaine altogether. But the idea of stopping marijuana, which I had used every day for the last 15 years, was ridiculous. And I had never had an alcohol problem, so there was no way that I was about to stop drinking.

George received a great deal of confrontation from other patients and the treatment staff about his denial, and he was surprised and dismayed to find so little interest in his "war stories," which glorified his drug use and dealing. After he had been in the hospital for several days, George's feelings began to change.

> As all of these drugs were getting out of my system, I realized that I hadn't had one straight day in at least 15 years. I began to like the way I was feeling. I could think more clearly, and I started to get off on being straight. I started meeting people from CA that I really respected—guys who had been on the streets and who were learning a different way of life.

George's wife was concurrently learning more about addiction and enabling behavior (see Chapter 6). When George initially considered leaving the hospital prematurely, she received support from other relatives and the treatment staff for her insistence that he stay in treatment.

In individual psychotherapy, George began to understand how he used drugs and drug dealing to try to make up for his feelings of low self-esteem. As he found other ways to feel good about himself, he began to feel less desperate about the prospect of a drug-free life:

> Even when I left the hospital, I had tremendous reservations about the idea of staying straight. That's why I really held on to the CA slogan that tells you to take things one day at a time. One day didn't seem all that hard. The other saying that I held on to for a long time was, "Fake it till you make it." I faked it for a long time, going through the motions of saying and doing all the right things. But now, one year later, I really believe that my life is much better than when I was using drugs. I don't have thousands of dollars coming into my hand every few days, but I don't have all that money going out, either. My mind is clear, my business is good, and even my marriage has been salvaged. What helped me most about going into the hospital was having people on my back every day, constantly confronting me, and being in an environment where I couldn't just take off and get high whenever I wanted to. What I learned from that experience was that I could survive bad feelings, which is something that I hadn't forced myself to do for 20 years.

Therapeutic communities. Therapeutic communities, sometimes known as *concept houses,* are self-help residential treatment programs that focus on the rehabilitation of certain subgroups of chronic drug users, particularly those who have failed in other treatment modalities. These highly confrontational programs, which are usually run by recovering addicts, are based on a theory that drug addiction occurs because of a combination of immature personality traits and because of an environment that never compels the individual to face up to reality. A therapeutic community seeks to reverse this process by forcing its residents to face frustrations and uncomfortable feelings without seeking an escape through drug use. These programs do so by creating a structured community that focuses on interpersonal concerns, particularly responsibility toward that community and the competent handling of aggression, hostility, and drug urges. Residents work their way up through the structured hierarchy of the community by demonstrating honesty and responsibility and by remaining drug free. Residents who do well in the system serve as role models for newcomers, and some graduates stay on to become staff members.

The highly confrontational nature of therapeutic communities, coupled with most addicts' ambivalence about seeking treatment, leads to a high dropout rate in these facilities. However, for those who stay in these programs, success rates on measures of drug abstinence and psychological maturity are relatively encouraging. Because therapeutic communities are stressful, psychologically difficult, long-term programs (they typically range from several months to two years in duration), they are usually not recommended as a first treatment effort. Rather, they are normally reserved for people who have failed at other treatment methods. The type of drug user who can benefit most from such a program tends to be someone with a chronic history of antisocial behavior or a longstanding record of poor vocational performance. For such individuals, the emphasis in therapeutic communities on honesty and responsibility can be quite beneficial.

The following example illustrates such a case: "Ed," a 24-year-old cocaine user, was referred to a therapeutic community after he had failed in his second attempt at outpatient treatment following hospitalization. Ed had abused numerous drugs and alcohol since age 13, with intravenous cocaine abuse predominating during the past two years. He had financed his habit through drug dealing and street crime, and he had been arrested several times for drug-related offenses. He had dropped out of school when he was 16 years old and had never worked for more than two consecutive months. Ed entered a therapeutic community reluctantly, but he found it quite helpful:

> When I was there, all distractions were taken away from me, and I had to look at myself honestly for the first time. Everyone else in there was as good a con artist as I was, so all of my attempts to get over on people didn't fly. I used to take pride in being the best sneak thief in my town, but now I'm beginning to feel good about myself for being honest. I also think that I'm able to help other people with drug problems because I understand so well how addicts think.

Ed was in a therapeutic community for one year. While there, he began working for his high school equivalency degree. When he obtained his degree, he joined the staff of the therapeutic community. He has been a highly respected employee in the community for the past year.

Halfway houses.   Halfway houses offer drug-dependent individuals the opportunity to live in a structured setting while getting involved in outpatient treatment and developing a life-style that does not revolve around drug use. Halfway houses are frequently helpful for people without solid living situations (e.g., people living with active substance users) who are about to be discharged from a drug treatment program. Because relapse rates for cocaine users tend to be highest in the period soon after discharge, a living situation supportive of abstinence is critical in helping individuals establish important life-style changes during this difficult early period. Some halfway houses will accept people from the community who can benefit from an improved living situation, but who do not require a full hospital program.

How to Choose the Right Type of Treatment

Many people who have cocaine problems are unsure about how to help themselves. As we can see by the large variety of treatment methods listed above, choosing the proper form of treatment can be quite difficult. For a cocaine user who may already be ambivalent about stopping his or her drug use, the confusion created by the multitude of different treatment techniques can offer a further excuse to put off seeking help at all.

The best way for a cocaine user to choose a proper treatment program is to talk with someone who is knowledgeable about cocaine abuse. Some people with cocaine problems can benefit by speaking with their personal physicians, who may have some expertise in the area of cocaine abuse or can refer them to the proper individual or local agency for a consultation. People who do not have a personal physician can call a well-known hospital in their area to ask for a cocaine or drug abuse specialist. They can also call their state medical or psychiatric society, or a local medical school, and ask for the name of someone who specializes in the treatment of cocaine or other substance abuse. Alternatively, they may make an appointment at a reputable drug abuse treatment program in the area. In the meantime, attending NA, AA, or CA meetings may be helpful in initiating treatment. The numbers for these organizations can be found in any local telephone directory.

Seven General Rules for Cocaine
Users Who Want to Quit

1: The Time to Stop Using Cocaine Is Now

Procrastination is one of the most frequent tactics of drug users in their relentless avoidance of treatment. "I'll quit tomorrow" is a euphemism for "I have no intention of quitting today."

2: You Should Stop All at Once, Not Gradually

Gradually cutting down on cocaine is a fruitless venture. Each use merely fuels the desire for more cocaine, and the recovery process is postponed indefinitely. Because cocaine withdrawal can cause depression, the drug should be stopped in a supportive setting.

3: Stop Using All Other Drugs of Abuse, Including Alcohol and Marijuana

This rule is frequently very difficult for cocaine users to accept. Perhaps alcohol and marijuana have never caused them any difficulties; they feel that they have a specific problem with cocaine, not with all drugs and alcohol. However, the use of alcohol or marijuana frequently represents an initial step toward relapse to cocaine. Because these drugs decrease inhibitions, one or two drinks may make a cocaine user feel somewhat less resolute about abstaining from cocaine than he or she feels while sober.

This phenomenon is illustrated by the following case example: "Ralph," a 33-year-old musician, was hospitalized because of cocaine abuse. He had been injecting cocaine intravenously every 15 minutes during the week before admission, causing serious abscesses on both arms. After being hospitalized for nine days, he was discharged to home with the recommendation that he refrain from all drugs and alcohol. At first, he followed this regimen successfully, and he was able to refuse two offers to use cocaine during this period. However, approximately two months after his discharge, Ralph went out to dinner and ordered a half bottle of wine, to share with his wife. This had been his customary drinking pattern before his hospitalization; he drank only on weekends at restaurants, and he rarely imbibed more than two glasses of wine in an evening. That night, he saw a former cocaine-using companion at the restaurant. This friend, who had offered him cocaine several weeks previously, repeated the offer on this evening, and Ralph accepted. He later said,

I had had two glasses of wine, and I wasn't drunk at all; I was just feeling good. At the time that he offered me the cocaine, I truly believed that one line wouldn't hurt me. I know that I wouldn't have made that same decision, though, if I had been stone cold sober.

Five days later, Ralph was again injecting cocaine every 15 minutes and was rehospitalized.

It is important to realize that in some cases, stopping drug use suddenly may cause potentially dangerous withdrawal symptoms (e.g., in the case of an individual who is drinking heavily and regularly). Thus one should consult with a physician before stopping any drug suddenly.

4: Change Your Life-Style

Cocaine users cannot associate with drug-using companions, nor can they safely frequent establishments (e.g., bars and clubs) in which alcohol and drug use are central activities. In Chapter 5, we discussed how craving increases during conditions that remind someone of his or her association with drugs. Thus cocaine users frequently have urges for the drug when they associate with fellow users, when they enter areas in which they had previously used drugs, and when they see drug-related paraphernalia (e.g, mirrors, razor blades, matches, straws, or needles). Because most follow-up studies of drug and alcohol users show that relapse is most common during the early stages of recovery, we advise that people to avoid such stimuli diligently, especially early in treatment (which leads to our next rule).

5: Whenever Possible, Avoid Situations, People, and Places That Cause Drug Urges

When it is impossible to avoid these situations, it is important to prepare for them in advance in order to be able to handle them safely. Cocaine users in recovery should avoid testing themselves to monitor how well they are doing. The phenomenon of testing one-self is quite common in drug users who are attempting to stop. They mistakenly believe that "passing a test" proves that their problem is well under control. A common assumption among those who challenge themselves is, "If I can survive this test, then I can get through anything, and I'll never use cocaine again." Unfortunately, nothing could be further from the truth.

For example, recovering cocaine users might test themselves by walking past their dealer's house to convince themselves that they do not need to go inside. Such behavior is likely to produce one of two unhappy results: they either fail the initial test by going inside the dealer's house, or they walk past the dealer's house and thereby become unafraid to do it again, thus becoming overconfident. Overconfidence leads to a loss of the self-vigilance that is necessary for ongoing recovery. If a drug user does not fear the ability to relapse, he or she is at high risk to fail. One of the implications of the "one day at a time" concept so frequently espoused at AA and similar groups is the fact that yesterday's abstinence does not ensure the same result today. Similarly, passing a test today does not mean that one will be able to resist drugs tomorrow. In fact, the resulting overconfidence from passing such a test may decrease the likelihood of remaining abstinent the next day. We therefore strongly advise people to avoid such tests.

6: Look for Other Rewards

Drug users frequently forget how to treat themselves well and enjoy themselves while drug free. They often ignore hobbies, stop exercising, eat badly, lose touch with drug-free friends, lose interest in sex, ignore their physical well-being, and lead a life generally devoid of chemical-free pleasure. Learning how to reconnect with the drug-free world will likely be one of the most difficult recovery tasks for many cocaine users; some may find that they have forgotten how to talk about anything except drugs. Self-help groups such as NA frequently hold social functions such as parties, dances, and sporting events to facilitate this process of reintegration. We also encourage our patients to reestablish relationships with old drug-free friends.

7: Take Good Care of Your Body: Eat Right and Exercise

Researchers at Fair Oaks Hospital in Summit, New Jersey, have found that vitamin deficiencies are quite common in chronic cocaine users. This is not surprising, because cocaine is an appetite suppressant. The resumption of normal eating habits can therefore be an important part of the overall recovery process. Regular exercise is also potentially helpful for cocaine users, who often allow themselves to get into poor physical condition. Exercise can also be used as a social activity and as a substitute for cocaine use during periods of high drug craving. Finally, strenuous exercise may help to decrease anxiety, perhaps through the release of opiate-like compounds in the brain called *endorphins;* the sense of well-being triggered by the release of these chemicals may decrease the desire for drugs.

Pathways to Recovery

There are many routes to recovery from cocaine abuse. Some individuals stop on their own, some go to self-help groups, some seek individual psychotherapy, and others require hospitalization. Despite the variety of specific treatment methods, it does appear that certain general factors may facilitate recovery in individuals who are dependent on cocaine or other drugs of abuse:

1. Individuals who have solid employment or school histories tend to fare better than those with erratic work records. Remaining drug free requires daily commitment and follow-through, which must be accomplished regardless of one's mood. These characteristics are also necessary to maintain a solid work re-

cord; those who are able to wake up and go to work on days when they do not feel like doing so are able to maintain better job histories than those who give in to their desire to go back to bed.

2. People who will experience a definite, immediate adverse consequence as the result of further cocaine use tend to do well in treatment. Thus the imminent fear of job loss, divorce, medical problems, or a jail term on resumption of cocaine use can provide a powerful incentive for recovery. The success of such threats depends on their credibility and the extent to which they will hurt the patient. This phenomenon is the theoretical basis for the "contingency contracting" treatment program (discussed above).

3. Another factor that is particularly helpful in the recovery of some substance users is the ability to find a new source of hope and self-esteem. This may come from religious involvement, self-help meetings, a helpful psychotherapy relationship, or a new love relationship uncontaminated by the difficulties brought about by the cocaine user's drug-related behavior.

Just as there are many pathways into cocaine abuse, there are many routes out. Although abstinence from cocaine does not guarantee happiness, study results thus far are encouraging: cocaine-dependent individuals who attain lasting recovery appear to experience greatly improved functioning in most other areas of their lives as well.

Chapter 9

Questions Frequently Asked About Cocaine

Questions Frequently Asked by the General Public

What is cocaine?
Cocaine is a stimulant drug derived from the South American coca plant, *Erythroxylon coca*. Its most important actions include stimulation of the central nervous system (the brain and spinal cord) and its ability to produce local anesthesia. *Cocaine hydrochloride* is the scientific name for the powdery white form of cocaine that is used intranasally or intravenously.

What is "crack?"
"Crack" is a form of cocaine that gives an intense "high" when smoked. Crack is produced by mixing cocaine hydrochloride with water and sodium bicarbonate (baking soda). This mixture is heated until all the water has evaporated. The resultant product consists of small chips containing alkaline cocaine that resemble white pebbles. These "rocks" can then be smoked, most typically in a pipe.

How much does cocaine cost?
Illicit ("street") cocaine costs about $50 to $100 a gram (1/28th of an ounce) in most metropolitan areas. Crack, which is usually sold in very small quantities, can be purchased for as little as $2 to $10

for a 50- to 100-milligram rock. Pharmaceutical (legal) cocaine costs only about $50 an ounce (or about $1.79 per gram).

Is cocaine addicting?

Yes. The American Psychiatric Association (APA) in its *Diagnostic and Statistical Manual of Mental Disorders, Fourth Edition* (DSM-IV) defines *substance dependence* (we use *dependence* as synonymous with *addiction*) as "a maladaptive pattern of substance use, leading to clinically significant impairment or distress, as manifested by three or more of the following occurring at any time in the same twleve-month period:" (the specific criteria used to make the diagnosis of cocaine dependence in DSM-IV are listed in Table 3; see Chapter 5). The APA's definition is echoed by the World Health Organization and the National Institute on Drug Abuse. It is clear that many cocaine users do lose control over their use and that they often use the drug despite adverse consequences. For years, the generally accepted medical definition of *addiction (dependence)* required the presence of one or both of the following two factors: tolerance to the drug (the need for increased intake to obtain the same drug effect) and physical signs of withdrawal after stopping drug use. Because abruptly stopping cocaine use does not cause dramatic medical symptoms, cocaine was long considered to be physically nonaddicting. The presence of tolerance and physical withdrawal are no longer considered to be the only two factors to define *addiction* or *drug dependence.*

Is crack more addicting than other forms of cocaine?

For most people, crack is more addicting than cocaine used intranasally. The characteristics of crack that make it so addictive include the intensity of the euphoria it produces, its nearly immediate onset of action, and the brevity of the high. In addition, the aftermath of smoking crack is often characterized by severe craving for more drug. Although some individuals may stop after limiting themselves to one or two "hits," repetitive use is a common pattern. Crack is considered approximately as addicting as intravenous cocaine, which has a similarly rapid onset of action and also produces an intense high.

Is cocaine an aphrodisiac?

Cocaine has certainly developed a reputation as a sexual stimulant. In fact, one of cocaine's nicknames is the "love drug." For some people, cocaine does initially stimulate sexual drive and enhance sexual pleasure. However, in a survey of regular cocaine users, only 13% of respondents experienced sexual stimulation from cocaine. Moreover, as cocaine use becomes more chronic and habitual, interest in sex and ability to perform often decreases, because the user's interest in anything other than cocaine diminishes.

Since cocaine use in this country is declining, is it still a major public health problem?

Although the absolute number of people using cocaine in this country has been decreasing since 1985, the number of individuals with serious cocaine problems, as measured by daily drug use, has actually increased. In addition, the number of cocaine-related emergencies and cocaine-related deaths has grown. The number of acquired immunodeficiency syndrome (AIDS) cases among intravenous cocaine users is also increasing. Thus there may be fewer people who use cocaine on an occasional basis, but more who have a serious addiction. Cocaine use therefore remains a serious public health problem in this country.

Questions Frequently Asked by Occasional Cocaine Users

Is it possible to overdose on cocaine?

Yes. In fact, the number of cocaine-related emergencies has been steadily increasing during the past decade. In a three-month period during 1991, the government's Drug Abuse Warning Network recorded more than 25,000 cocaine related emergencies. Similarly, cocaine-related deaths have been increasing. In 1991, more than 3,000 people died from cocaine overdose—a sixfold increase over 1985. The major causes of death from cocaine overdose include 1) irregular heartbeat leading to cardiac arrest, 2) extremely high blood pressure that can cause bleeding into the brain (cerebral hemorrhage), 3) continuous epileptic seizures (status epilepticus), and 4) respiratory arrest.

Is it possible to overdose from snorting cocaine?
Yes. Many cocaine users incorrectly believe that snorting cocaine is "safe." Although crack smoking and intravenous cocaine use are medically more dangerous than intranasal use, snorting cocaine offers no guarantee against overdose. Overdoses are unpredictable; there is no single "lethal" dose of cocaine. Rather, each individual is vulnerable to overdose after a different amount of drug intake. A dose of cocaine that may barely affect one user may be fatal for another. Moreover, an overdose may occur during initial "experimentation" with the drug or after long-term use. Another hazard of cocaine, regardless of the route of administration, is the fact that buying cocaine on the street is truly a blind purchase. You can never be sure exactly how much pure cocaine you are buying and how much adulterant ("cut") you are being sold. Therefore, if you are accustomed to buying highly adulterated cocaine and you are sold a batch of relatively pure cocaine, you may have a very serious reaction to the same amount of powder, which contains a much larger dose of cocaine.

I know that smoking crack or using intravenous cocaine can be very addicting, but is it possible to get addicted to cocaine just by snorting?
Yes. Most studies have shown that a significant percentage of the people being treated for chronic cocaine abuse are exclusively intranasal users. Thus "just" snorting offers no protection against cocaine-related problems. An additional hazard of intranasal use is the risk of progression to other, more dangerous forms of cocaine abuse. Most intravenous users and freebase smokers began by snorting cocaine. Many of these people had previously assured themselves that they would never resort to these more hazardous forms of use. However, heavy cocaine use can alter previously solid judgment. Chronic users may become bolder and more careless, and they may take chances with their health that would previously have been unthinkable.

I am an occasional cocaine snorter, and I sometimes sell small amounts of cocaine to friends. How much legal trouble can I get into for this?

Possession of cocaine for any purpose other than legitimate medical use is illegal. Although cocaine possession is frequently classified as a misdemeanor, the sale of cocaine is generally considered a felony. Moreover, many states do not set a minimum amount of cocaine that needs to be sold to be considered drug trafficking. Enforcement of these laws varies from state to state and from judge to judge. Thus the penalty for a first offense of cocaine possession may vary from a slap on the wrist to 20 years in prison. Penalties for the sale of cocaine may depend on the amount sold. However, in some states, a first arrest for the sale of any amount of cocaine may be punishable by up to 99 years in prison.

Although I don't think I have a cocaine problem, I know that drug users are usually the last ones to know (or admit) that they have a problem. How would I know if I did have a cocaine problem?

If cocaine causes problems in your life, you have a cocaine problem. Thus if the use of cocaine directly or indirectly leads to difficulties in your work, school, or relationships or if it creates financial, medical, psychological, or legal difficulties, you have a cocaine problem. In addition, if your cocaine use has led you to behave in ways that you would have previously considered unacceptable, then you have a cocaine problem. Many people find that the initial symptom of a cocaine problem is preoccupation with the drug; they spend an increasing amount of time thinking about the drug, thus diminishing the amount of energy they have to devote to other activities. A self-test for cocaine dependence can be found in the Appendix.

However, even if you feel that your cocaine use is not currently a problem, there is still good reason to stop. Continued use is likely to result in increasingly difficult problems, along with the significant risk of developing cocaine dependence. The surest way to avoid these consequences is to stop all cocaine use while you feel that your use is controllable. If you do try to stop and find that you are not able to, we urge you to seek professional help.

I'm thinking of getting pregnant, and I like to snort cocaine. Should I give up the drug while I'm pregnant? How about while I'm nursing?
It is generally a good idea to avoid all drugs while you are pregnant. Recent evidence has underscored this point with regard to cocaine. Although still under study, the following adverse effects of cocaine use during pregnancy have been reported: premature birth, low birth weight, and increased risk of deformities of the genital and urinary organs. After birth, "crib death," or sudden unexplained death, may be more likely in babies exposed to cocaine in utero. Children whose mothers used cocaine also have a high rate of behavioral difficulties including hypersensitivity, irritability, and difficulty forming relationships. These children tend to do poorly in school and often have learning disabilities. As for nursing, small amounts of cocaine have been detected in the breast milk of nursing mothers. Therefore, the use of cocaine by a woman who is breast-feeding directly exposes her baby to the toxic effects of the cocaine.

Can you get hepatitis just from snorting cocaine?
Yes. Hepatitis B and hepatitis C are transmitted via the blood and via intimate sexual contact. Although sharing needles provides the most frequent route of transmission from one person to another, sharing snorting paraphernalia may similarly spread the disease. A microscopic drop of blood from a straw, dollar bill, or "tooter" is sufficient to transmit the virus.

Can you get hepatitis more than once?
Yes. Although many people become immune after being exposed to hepatitis B, this does not confer immunity to hepatitis C. A relapse of hepatitis can also be precipitated by drinking alcohol, which has a direct toxic effect on the liver.

Can you get AIDS from using cocaine?
Yes. Intravenous drug users are one of the groups at highest risk of contracting AIDS, a deadly disease that attacks the immune system. Moreover, the use of cocaine (frequently along with other drugs) may impair judgment and increase the likelihood of engaging in

risky sexual encounters, which may lead to human immunodeficiency virus (HIV) infection.

I find that I don't enjoy cocaine as much as I used to. In fact, I get depressed and anxious on the drug. But I find myself using more in an attempt to reexperience the great highs that I used to get. What's wrong?

You are describing the typical symptoms of the transition from occasional cocaine use to compulsive use. If you do not stop, you appear to be headed for trouble. Initially, most occasional cocaine users experience euphoria from the drug. However, as continued use becomes more frequent and intensive, users tend to feel the opposite of euphoria; depression, anxiety, and irritability are common reactions. Many individuals respond as you did: they take more cocaine in an attempt to reexperience the euphoria. Unfortunately, the next stage in the progression of this pattern is generally characterized by paranoia, often accompanied by frightening hallucinations. The time for you to stop your cocaine use is now. If you cannot do it on your own, you should seek help immediately.

Questions Frequently Asked by People Dependent on Cocaine

I know a lot of people who can snort one or two lines of cocaine and put it down. But, regardless of how much cocaine is around, I'll use it until it's gone. Why can some people use the drug with control while others can't?

There is no simple answer to this question. Many researchers are trying to determine what makes some people particularly vulnerable to cocaine addiction. Most experts believe that a combination of factors leads to addiction, including the user's response to cocaine, the availability of the drug, and life circumstances. For example, some research, including our own, has found an increased rate of mood disorders among chronic cocaine users. This has led to speculation that a history of depression or mood swings might increase one's risk for cocaine addiction. However, addiction cannot occur without drug availability, including a means to pay it or a willingness to engage in illegal activities to do so. It is important to keep in mind that no one starts out as a cocaine addict. Many people start out as "controlled users." However, some occasional users become addicted. Unfortunately, there is no way to predict ahead of time who will become dependent and who will not.

My cocaine use is out of control. I want to cut back to social use again. Any suggestions?
Once you have become dependent on cocaine, the only way to regain control over your life is to try to stop all drug use completely. The path to cocaine addiction at some point be comes a one-way street, in which the route back to occasional use is blocked. Virtually everyone who enters treatment because of cocaine abuse has already tried to "cut back" dozens of times. Unfortunately, many of these individuals inflict a great deal of damage on themselves and others before giving up on this approach. Therefore, your goal should be complete abstinence, not controlled drug use.

I was recently treated for cocaine abuse and was told that I not only have to give up cocaine, but all other drugs, including marijuana. They even want me to stop drinking. I've never had a problem with any other drugs, and I don't even like the taste of alcohol much. My only problem was with cocaine. Isn't the recommendation to give up other drugs and alcohol a little excessive?
Although many patients balk at our recommendation for complete abstinence from all drugs of abuse (including alcohol), we feel that this advice is sound. Using other drugs presents two risks for you. First, you may become dependent on the other drug. For example, 60% of the cocaine users admitted to our unit use three or more drugs regularly, and more than half are alcoholic. An aversion to the taste of alcohol unfortunately offers you no protection against the future development of alcoholism. A second hazard of alcohol or other drug use is the fact that even low doses of most drugs will decrease your inhibitions. Thus even a relatively small amount of alcohol or marijuana may make you feel less committed to total ab-

stinence from cocaine than you felt while completely sober. We have seen a large number of cocaine users return to cocaine use after having just one or two drinks. Resolve, willpower, good judgment, and the best of intentions are all soluble in alcohol. If cocaine is available after you have had a couple of drinks, you may decide that "one line won't hurt," although you would know better while completely sober.

I am beginning to have trouble falling asleep after using cocaine, and I've been drinking more and using Valium to help me sleep. Should I worry about this?

Yes. More than half of the patients admitted to our treatment unit are also alcoholic, and some have problems with sedative-hypnotic drugs such as Valium. The use of other drugs to mitigate the stimulant effects of cocaine or to buffer the symptoms of a cocaine "crash" is very common and quite dangerous. Moreover, the combination of cocaine and alcohol may lead to serious medical complications. Unfortunately, dependence on sedative-hypnotic drugs or alcohol frequently continues even after the cocaine abuse has stopped.

I'm worried about my cocaine use. How do I go about finding help?

Admitting that you have a problem is an important first step. The types of treatment available for cocaine abuse vary in their approach, intensity, and cost. In Chapter 8 of this book we described the various types of treatment methods that are available for cocaine users. If you are not sure which route to take, it would be helpful for you to consult someone in your area who is knowledgeable about cocaine abuse. That person will be best able to recommend a course of treatment for you. To find such a person, there are several paths you can take:

1. Ask your physician if he or she knows a knowledgeable person whom you can consult about the problem.
2. Call your state psychiatric or medical society and ask for the name of a person who specializes in drug dependence. Then try to make an appointment with that person.

3. Call a local medical school and ask for the name of the person who runs their drug abuse program or who teaches at the school about drug abuse. If that person cannot see you, he or she will be able to refer you to someone else knowledgeable in the field.
4. If you know of a good drug abuse program in your area, call the director and ask for a consultation or a referral.
5. In addition to one of these steps, you can call your local chapter of Narcotics Anonymous, Cocaine Anonymous, Alcoholics Anonymous, Rational Recovery, or Women for Sobriety and start attending their meetings.

Can psychotherapy help me to stop using cocaine?
There is no single form of treatment that will help every cocaine user. Psychotherapy, like all treatment approaches for cocaine abuse, is extremely valuable for some people and less effective in helping others to stop their cocaine use. Although abstinence is a common goal of virtually all forms of treatment, the approaches leading to this endpoint vary considerably. Some people benefit primarily from attending self-help groups such as Narcotics Anonymous, Cocaine Anonymous, Alcoholics Anonymous, or Rational Recovery. For others, certain medications may prove very useful. In some cases, hospitalization may be required to stop cocaine use. Conversely, there are cocaine-dependent individuals who have simply stopped on their own with no outside help. If you have questions about whether individual psychotherapy would be helpful for you, we suggest talking with someone who is knowledgeable about both drug abuse and psychotherapy. This person may be able to advise you about the treatment approach that would most likely be helpful.

Does cocaine abuse run in families?
Because cocaine abuse has been common in the United States only since the early 1970s, there is little information about the transmission of the problem from generation to generation. We will have to wait until the next century before we will have the answer to this question.

Questions Frequently Asked by People Who Treat Cocaine Users

When do you recommend hospitalization for a cocaine user?
This is an area of some controversy. In general, the decision whether to hospitalize a patient is made on the basis of the severity of the patient's current condition. There are several signs that would lead us to initially recommend hospitalization for a cocaine user: 1) suicidal or homicidal thoughts, 2) reckless behavior that is placing the patient or others in danger, 3) dependence on alcohol or another drug that requires detoxification, or 4) concurrent medical or psychiatric illness that would make outpatient treatment untenable. If a cocaine user does not meet any of these criteria, we ordinarily recommend outpatient treatment initially. For patients who are unsuccessful in outpatient treatment, more intensive treatment, including hospitalization, may be recommended as a backup plan.

I have read some very impressive statistics supporting certain treatments for cocaine abuse, such as desipramine and contingency contracting. Do you recommend using these methods for all cocaine users?
There is no single "best" treatment for all cocaine users (see Chapter 8). There are clearly some individuals for whom contingency contracting is extremely useful. However, there are other patients who will relapse despite such a contingency program and may then be worse off for having made such a contract. Thus this form of treatment should only be offered after carefully evaluating the patient's total life circumstances and discussing the pros and cons of the treatment with the patient. Although some of the early work on the use of the antidepressant drug desipramine in cocaine users was encouraging, more recent studies have been rather disappointing. Perhaps this is partly related to the fact that the onset of action of the drug may take two weeks or more, which is often the time cocaine users are vulnerable to relapse. In any event, desipramine, like other forms of treatment, is not a panacea for cocaine abuse.

However, it may be helpful for a certain segment of the cocaine-abusing population–particularly those individuals with coexisting mood disorders.

Do you recommend urine screening for cocaine users in the hospital?
Absolutely. Because it is difficult for even experienced treatment personnel to detect cocaine use clinically, there is no substitute for urine screening as an instrument of detection and deterrence. For urine screening to be effective, however, the testing must be random, supervised, and accurate.

Do different laboratory techniques vary in their ability to detect cocaine in the urine accurately?
Yes. The best laboratory methodology for detecting cocaine use uses an enzyme immunoassay (EIA) technique such as Enzyme Multiplied Immunoassay Technique (EMIT), with confirmation of positive results by combined gas chromatography-mass spectrometry (GC-MS). Thin-layer chromatography (TLC), which is used in many laboratories, is less useful, because it can detect cocaine or its metabolite benzoylecgonine in urine for only about 12 to 24 hours after cocaine use.

How long does cocaine or its metabolites stay in the urine?
EIA techniques such as EMIT can detect the cocaine metabolite benzoylecgonine for up to 48 hours after drug use. GC-MS ordinarily can detect benzoylecgonine in the urine for several days after drug use, though we have occasionally seen positive urine screens in very heavy cocaine users for longer periods after cocaine use.

Questions Frequently Asked by
Family Members of Cocaine Users

I have just found out that my son is addicted to cocaine. Did I do something wrong during his childhood that could have caused his drug problem?

This is one of the questions most commonly asked by parents of cocaine users. Frequently those who do not ask are reluctant to do so because they are afraid that they already know the answer. The answer, however, is not simple because there is no single "cause" of cocaine abuse. There is good evidence, for instance, that childhood trauma cannot be blamed as a cause of alcoholism. Although research on cocaine abuse is comparatively new, no studies have shown that specific childhood experiences or family interactions predispose an individual to the future development of cocaine abuse.

How can I tell if my teenage daughter is using cocaine?

If your daughter is using the drug frequently, you may notice a disturbance in her sleeping pattern, with late nights followed by daytime somnolence; she may be particularly moody and irritable; she may have frequent "cold" symptoms; she may lose weight rapidly; and she is likely to borrow (or steal) money from you frequently. She may develop problems in school, and she may leave the house for long periods of time without explanation. These symptoms, in addition to an attitude of secretiveness and distrust, may be warning signs of cocaine use. However, it may be very difficult to detect cocaine use, particularly in its early stages. Therefore, it is important to keep the lines of communication open with your daughter and to have frank discussions with her about drugs.

My husband has just entered treatment for cocaine abuse. What are the chances of his recovery?

Although cocaine dependence is a chronic illness with the potential for relapse always present, it is treatable. Although treatment outcome studies are in their preliminary stages, early results have been quite promising. Recovery from cocaine addiction, however, is a long-term process that involves hard work and sacrifices. It can be particularly difficult for family members when the recovering user devotes a great deal of time and energy to treatment activities. Therefore, it is often helpful for family members to seek support of their own, such as individual therapy, Nar-Anon, or a similar support group.

I think my wife is addicted to cocaine. I have talked with her constantly about stopping, but it does no good. This drug is ruining our marriage, our kids, and our finances. But she keeps claiming that it's "no big deal." How can she keep saying this and what can I do?

You have provided a vivid illustration of why addiction is often called a "disease of denial." It is this denial or minimization of the wreckage caused by drug abuse that makes living with an addicted person so painful and exasperating. It is your wife's illness of addiction that keeps her from seeing what cocaine is doing to her. She clearly needs treatment, and you may be able to help her get it. The best way to help her is to confront her with the consequences of her cocaine abuse in a clear, nonjudgmental, but firm manner. If your children are old enough to do so, you may involve them in the confrontation as well. The details of such an encounter, called an *intervention,* are described in Chapter 6. You must also think about what you will do if your wife does not accept treatment, because you must not allow yourself and the rest of your family to be destroyed by your wife's addiction. To obtain guidance and support during this process, we suggest that you speak with someone in a drug abuse treatment center who is experienced in performing family interventions. You might also find Nar-Anon meetings helpful, whereas your children may benefit from Alateen meetings if they are old enough. If your wife does enter treatment, we urge you to participate in the part of the program for family members, because the illness of addiction affects the entire family.

Self-Test for Cocaine Dependence

The following self-test consists of a list of questions designed to examine your use of cocaine and to identify the potential problems that the drug can cause. The questions are organized around the types of difficulties that are most frequently associated with cocaine use. Answer the questions honestly; there are no right or wrong answers. If you find yourself answering "yes" to even a few of the questions, you may have a significant cocaine problem, warranting serious attention. For advice on how to seek help, see Chapter 8.

+ Medical problems
  1. Do you frequently have "cold" symptoms, nasal congestion, or nosebleeds?
  2. Have you ever had a seizure (convulsion) as the result of cocaine use?
  3. Have you ever had a frightening physical experience while on cocaine, such as severe heart palpitations or a feeling that you were in serious medical danger?
  4. Have you ever used cocaine intravenously?
  5. Have you ever used the same needle more than once?
  6. Have you ever shared needles with other drug users?
  7. Have you ever shared needles with other drug users that you suspected had hepatitis?

8. Have you ever shared needles with other drug users that you suspected had AIDS?

9. Have you ever had shortness of breath, difficulty breathing, or a serious cough as the result of freebasing or smoking crack?

+ Psychological problems
    1. Do you continue using cocaine despite the fact that it makes you anxious? Jittery? Irritable? Restless? Belligerent?
    2. Have you ever hallucinated while on cocaine?
    3. Did the use of cocaine ever make you feel that there were people trying to harm you when in fact you know that they weren't?
    4. Do you get depressed ("crash") when you stop using?
    5. Do you use more cocaine to end the crash?
    6. Do you use other drugs or alcohol to treat some of the undesirable effects of cocaine, such as insomnia, anxiety, depression, or restlessness?

+ Problems with other people
    1. Do other people complain about your cocaine use?
    2. Do you find that you are choosing cocaine over the company of other people?
    3. Do you use cocaine primarily when you are alone?
    4. Has cocaine caused a lack of sexual interest?
    5. Has cocaine impaired your ability to perform sexually?
    6. Have you found yourself lying, cheating, manipulating, or stealing from your friends or relatives because of your cocaine use?
    7. Are you more irritable and curt around other people?
    8. Have you found that an increasing number of your "friends" are drug-related acquaintances?
    9. Have you ever lost an important relationship because of your cocaine use?
    10. Do you find that more and more of your conversations are focusing on cocaine, to the exclusion of other topics that used to interest you?

Self-Test for Cocaine Dependence

+ Problems at work or school
  1. Do you get high at work or during school hours?
  2. Has your work or school performance declined as your use of cocaine has increased?
  3. Do you sometimes miss work or school either because you are high or because you are crashing?
  4. Do you believe that you would be doing better at work or school if you did not use cocaine?

+ Financial problems
  1. Has your use of cocaine ever caused financial problems?
  2. Have you ever spent money on cocaine that had been earmarked for something else?
  3. Have you ever stolen money or anything else in order to pay for cocaine?
  4. Have you ever "borrowed" money for cocaine and not paid it back?
  5. Have you ever sold cocaine in order to finance your own drug use?
  6. Has your income decreased because of poor business decisions made while intoxicated or in haste because you wanted to get high?
  7. Have you ever lamented the amount of money you have spent on cocaine?

+ Legal problems
  1. Have you ever been arrested for cocaine use?
  2. Have you ever driven a car while under the influence of cocaine?
  3. Have you ever performed illegal acts to obtain cocaine?

+ Loss of control, preoccupation, changing priorities
  1. Have you ever told yourself that you would stop cocaine immediately, then changed your mind and pledged to stop the next day?
  2. Do you find yourself constantly thinking about cocaine?
  3. Do you dream about cocaine?

4. Do you get an urge to use cocaine when you are exposed to people, places, or things (e.g., mirrors or razor blades) that remind you of the drug?

5. Have you become extremely discouraged by your unsuccessful attempts to stop using cocaine?

6. Have you ever thought about suicide because of your fear that you will never be able to stop using cocaine?

7. Do you feel that you have lost a sense of right and wrong since you started using cocaine?

8. Do you find yourself justifying your behavior to yourself when you would have clearly seen this behavior as immoral or wrong before you started using cocaine?

9. Do you feel that you have to use cocaine if it is around?

10. Do you use whatever amount of cocaine is available (i.e., do you use it until it is gone)?

11. Do you use cocaine even after telling yourself that you won't?

12. Do you think you have a problem with cocaine?

13. Do you think that you are dependent on cocaine?

Bibliography

AA World Services: Alcoholics Anonymous, 3rd Edition. New York, AA World Services, 1976

AA World Services: Twelve Steps and Twelve Traditions. New York, AA World Services, 1980

Ambre JJ, Belknap SM, Nelson J, et al: Acute tolerance to cocaine in humans. Clinical Pharmacology and Therapeutics 44:1–8, 1988

American Psychiatric Association: DSM-IV Draft Criteria: 3/1/93. Washington, DC, American Psychiatric Association, 1993

Begleiter H, Porjesz B: Potential biological markers in individuals at high risk for developing alcoholism. Alcoholism: Clinical and Experimental Research 12:488–494, 1988

Blume SB, Lesieur HR: Pathological gambling in cocaine abusers, in Cocaine. Edited by Washton AM, Gold MS. New York, Guilford, 1987, pp 208–213

Brody SL, Slovis CM, Wrenn KD: Cocaine-related medical problems: consecutive series of 233 patients. American Journal of Medicine 88:325–331, 1990

Brown E, Prager J, Lee HY, et al: CNS complications of cocaine abuse: prevalence, pathophysiology, and neuroradiology. American Journal of Roentgenology 159:137–147, 1992

Byck R: Cocaine Papers: Sigmund Freud. New York, Stonehill Publishing, 1974

Cadoret RJ, Troughton E, Gorman TW, et al: An adoption study of genetic and environmental factors in drug abuse. Archives of General Psychiatry 43:1131–1136, 1986

Carroll KM, Rounsaville BJ, Gawin FH: A comparative trial of psychotherapies for ambulatory cocaine abusers: relapse prevention and interpersonal therapy. American Journal of Drug and Alcohol Abuse 17:229–247, 1991

Carroll KM, Rounsaville BJ, Keller DS: Relapse prevention strategies for the treatment of cocaine abuse. American Journal of Drug and Alcohol Abuse 17:249–265, 1991

Chaisson RE, Bacchetti P, Osmond D, et al: Cocaine use and HIV infection in intravenous drug users in San Francisco. Journal of the American Medical Association 261:561–565, 1989

Chasnoff IJ: Cocaine and pregnancy: clinical and methodologic issues. Clinics in Perinatology 18:113–123, 1991

Chasnoff IJ, MacGregor S, Chisum G: Cocaine use during pregnancy: adverse perinatal outcome, in Problems of Drug Dependence, 1987: Proceedings of the 49th Annual Scientific Meeting, Committee on Problems of Drug Dependence, Inc. Edited by Harris L. Washington, DC, National Institute on Drug Abuse Research (Monograph 81), 1988, p 265

Chiu TTW, Vaughn AJ, Carzoli RP: Hospital costs for cocaine-exposed infants. Journal of the Florida Medical Association 77:897–900, 1990

Cloninger CR, Sigvardsson S, Bohman M: Childhood personality predicts alcohol abuse in young adults. Alcoholism: Clinical and Experimental Research 12:494–505, 1988

Cocaine use may be underestimated: high rate among arrested suspects casts doubt on US survey. The Washington Post, March 28, 1990, p A7

Conway JP: Significant others need help, too: alcoholism treatment is just as important to the rest of the family. Focus on Alcohol and Drug Issues 4:17–19, 1981

Cregler LL, Mark H: Special report: Medical complications of cocaine abuse. New England Journal of Medicine 315:1495–1500, 1986

Europe's cocaine epidemic. Wall Street Journal, November 16, 1990, p 12

Forrester JM, Steele AW, Waldron JA, et al: Crack lung: an acute pulmonary syndrome with a spectrum of clinical and histopathologic findings. American Review of Respiratory Diseases 142:462–467, 1990

Gawin FH: Cocaine addiction: psychology and neurophysiology. Science 251:1580–1586, 1991

Gawin FH, Kleber HD: Abstinence symptomatology and psychiatric diagnosis in cocaine abusers. Archives of General Psychiatry 43:107–113, 1986

Gawin FH, Kleber HD, Byck R, et al: Desipramine facilitation of initial cocaine abstinence. Archives of General Psychiatry 46:117–120, 1989

Goldfrank LR, Hoffman RS: The cardiovascular effects of cocaine. Annals of Emergency Medicine 20:165–173, 1991

Bibliography

Gust SW, Walsh JM: Research on the prevalence, impact, and treatment of drug abuse in the workplace. National Institute on Drug Abuse Research Monograph 100:3–24, 1991

Heroin is making comeback in lethal tandem with crack. New York Times, July 21, 1990, p 1

Higgins ST, Delaney DD, Budney AJ, et al: A behavioral approach to achieving initial cocaine abstinence. American Journal of Psychiatry 148:1218–1224, 1991

Holland RW, Marx JA, Earnest MP, et al: Grand mal seizures temporally related to cocaine use: clinical and diagnostic features. Annals of Emergency Medicine 21:772–776, 1992

Honer WG, Gewirtz G, Turey M: Psychosis and violence in cocaine smokers (letter). Lancet 2:451, 1987

In a crack house: dinner and drugs on the stove. The New York Times, April 6, 1991, p 1

Isner JM, Estes M, Thompson PD, et al: Acute cardiac events temporarily related to cocaine abuse. New England Journal of Medicine 315:1438–1443, 1986

Javaid JI, Fischman MW, Schuster CR, et al: Cocaine plasma concentration: relation to physiological and subjective effects in humans. Science 202:227–228, 1978

Jeri FR, Sanchez C, Del Dozo T: The syndrome of coca paste: observations in a group of patients in the Lima area. Journal of Psychoactive Drugs 10:361–370, 1978

Johanson CE, Fischman MW: The pharmacology of cocaine related to its abuse. Pharmacological Reviews 41:3–52, 1989

Jones RT: Marijuana-induced "high": influence of expectations, setting and previous drug experience. Pharmacological Review 23:359–369, 1971

Karan LD, Haller DL, Schnoll SH: Cocaine, in Clinical Textbook of Addictive Disorders. Edited by Frances RJ, Miller SI. New York, Guilford, 1991, pp 121–145

Kellerman JL: A Guide for the Family of the Alcoholic. New York, Al-Anon Family Group Headquarters, 1979

Khantzian EJ: The self-medication hypothesis of addictive disorders: focus on heroin and cocaine dependence. American Journal of Psychiatry 142:1259–1264, 1985

Kleber HD: Tracking the cocaine epidemic: The Drug Abuse Warning Network. Journal of the American Medical Association 26:2272–2273, 1991

Koob GF, Weiss F: Neuropharmacology of cocaine and ethanol dependence. Recent Developments in Alcoholism 10:201–233, 1992

Kosten TR: Neurobiology of abused drugs: opioids and stimulants. The Journal of Nervous and Mental Disease 178:217–227, 1990

Kosten TR: Pharmacotherapeutic interventions for cocaine abuse: matching patients to treatments. The Journal of Nervous and Mental Disease 177:379–389, 1989

Lehman WEK, Simpson DP: Patterns of drug use in a large metropolitan work force. National Institute on Drug Abuse Research Monograph 100:45–62, 1991

Louie AK, Lannon RA, Ketter TA: Treatment of cocaine-induced panic disorder. The American Journal of Psychiatry 146:40–44, 1989

Marzuk PM, Tardiff K, Leon AC, et al: Prevalence of recent cocaine use among motor vehicle fatalities in New York City. Journal of the American Medical Association 263:250–256, 1990

Marzuk PM, Tardiff K, Leon AC, et al: Prevalence of cocaine use among residents of New York City who committed suicide during a one-year period. American Journal of Psychiatry 149:371–375, 1992

Miller NS, Gold MS, Belkin BM, et al: Family history and diagnosis of alcohol dependence in cocaine dependence. Psychiatric Research 29:113–121, 1989

Mirin SM, Weiss RD, Michael J: Psychopathology in substance abusers: diagnosis and treatment. American Journal of Drug and Alcohol Abuse 14:139–157, 1988

Mirin SM, Weiss RD, Greenfield SF: Psychoactive substance use disorders, in The Practitioner's Guide to Psychoactive Drugs, 3rd Edition. Edited by Gelenberg AJ, Bassuk EL, Schoonover SC. New York, Plenum, 1991, pp 219–316

Mody CK, Miller BL, McIntyre HB, et al: Neurologic complications of cocaine abuse. Neurology 38:1189–1193, 1988

National Institute on Drug Abuse: National Household Survey on Drug Abuse 1991. Rockville, MD, National Clearinghouse for Drug Abuse Information, 1992

National Institute on Drug Abuse, Division of Epidemiology and Prevention Research: Drug Abuse Warning Network (DAWN) Files. Rockville, MD, U.S. Department of Health and Human Services, 1991

Nelson C: Styles of Enabling in the Codependents of Cocaine Abusers. San Diego, CA, United States International University, 1984

Noble EP, Blum K, Ritchie T, et al: Allelic association of the D2 dopamine receptor gene with receptor-binding characteristics in alcoholism. Archives of General Psychiatry 48:648–654, 1991

O'Brien CP, Childress AR, McLellan AT: Conditioning factors may help to understand and prevent relapse in patients who are recovering from drug dependence. National Institute on Drug Abuse Research Monograph 106:293–311, 1991

Om A, Warner M, Sabri, et al: Frequency of coronary artery disease and left ventricle dysfunction in cocaine users. American Journal of Cardiology 69:1549–1552, 1992

O'Malley S, Adamse M, Heaton RK, et al: Neuropsychological impairment in chronic cocaine abusers. The American Journal of Drug and Alcohol Abuse 18:131–144, 1992

Perez-Reyes M, DiGuiseppi S, Ondrusek G, et al: Freebase cocaine smoking. Clinical Pharmacology and Therapeutics 32:459–465, 1982

Pert A, Post R, Weiss SRB: Conditioning as a critical determinant of sensitization induced by psychomotor stimulants. National Institute on Drug Abuse Research Monograph 95:208–235, 1989

Post RM: Cocaine psychoses: a continuum model. American Journal of Psychiatry 132:225–231, 1975

Post RM, Kotin J, Goodwin FR: The effects of cocaine on depressed patients. American Journal of Psychiatry 131:511–517, 1974

Post RM, Weiss SRB: Psychomotor stimulant vs. local anesthetic effects of cocaine: role of behavioral sensitization and kindling. National Institute on Drug Abuse Research Monograph 88:217–238, 1988

Rawson RA, Obert JL, McCann MJ, et al: Cocaine treatment outcome: cocaine use following inpatient, outpatient, and no treatment, in Problems of Drug Dependence, 1985: Proceedings of the 47th Annual Scientific Meeting, Committee on Problems of Drug Dependence, Inc. Edited by Harris L. Washington, DC, National Institute on Drug Abuse Research (Monograph 67), 1986, pp 271–277

Resnick RB, Kestenbaum RS, Schwartz LK: Acute systemic effects of cocaine in man: a controlled study by intranasal and intravenous routes. Science 195:696–698, 1977

Roman PM: The use of EAPs in dealing with drug abuse in the workplace. National Institute on Drug Abuse Research Monograph 91:223–234, 1991

Rounsaville BJ, Anton SF, Carroll K, et al: Psychiatric diagnosis of treatment-seeking cocaine abusers. Archives of General Psychiatry 48:43–51, 1991

Rowbotham MC, Lowenstein DH: Neurologic consequences of cocaine use. Annual Review of Medicine 41:417–422, 1990

Satel SL, Edell WS: Cocaine-induced paranoia and psychosis proneness. American Journal of Psychiatry 148:1708–1711, 1991

Satel SL, Price LH, Palumbo JM, et al: Clinical phenomenology and neurobiology of cocaine abstinence: a prospective inpatient study. American Journal of Psychiatry 148:1712–1716, 1991

Satel SL, Southwick SM, Gawin FH: Clinical features of cocaine-induced paranoia. American Journal of Psychiatry 148(4):495–498, 1991

Schneider RJ, Khantzian EJ: Psychotherapy and patient needs in the treatment of alcohol and cocaine abuse. Recent Developments in Alcoholism 10:179–191, 1992

Schroeder EP: Legal aspects of urine screening. National Institute on Drug Abuse Research Monograph 95:218–224, 1989

Schuckit M: Subjective responses to alcohol in sons of alcoholics and control subjects. Archives of General Psychiatry 41:879–884, 1984

Schulamith L, Straussner A, Weinstein DL, et al: Effects of alcoholism on the family system. Health and Social Work 4:111–127, 1979

Shannon E: A losing battle. Time, December 3, 1990, pp 44–48

Shannon E: New kings of coke. Time, July 1, 1991, pp 29–33

Shannon M: Clinical toxicity of cocaine adulterants. Annals of Emergency Medicine 17:1243–1247, 1988

Sherer MA: Intravenous cocaine: psychiatric effects, biologic mechanisms. Biological Psychiatry 24:865–885, 1988

Siegel RK: Cocaine hallucinations. American Journal of Psychiatry 135:309–314, 1978

Slutsker L: Risks associated with cocaine use during pregnancy. Obstetrics and Gynecology 79(5):778–779, 1992

Smart RG: Crack cocaine use: a review of prevalence and adverse effects. American Journal of Drug and Alcohol Abuse 17:13–26, 1991

Steinberg MA, Kosten TA, Rounsaville BJ: Cocaine abuse and pathological gambling. American Journal on Addictions 1:121–132, 1992

Tannenbaum JH, Miller F: Electrocardiographic evidence of myocardial injury in psychiatrically hospitalized cocaine abusers. General Hospital Psychiatry 14:201–203, 1992

Teller DW, Devenyi P: Bromocriptine in cocaine withdrawal: does it work? International Journal of the Addictions 23:1197–1205, 1988

Tousexis A: Innocent victims. Time, May 13, 1991, pp 56–63

Vaillant GE: The Natural History of Alcoholism: Causes, Patterns and Paths to Recovery. Cambridge, MA, Harvard University Press, 1983

Van Dyke C, Barash PG, Jatlow P, et al: Cocaine: plasma concentrations after intranasal applications in man. Science 191:859–861, 1976

Verebey K, Gold MS: From coca leaves to crack: the effects of dose and routes of administration in abuse liability. Psychiatric Annals 18:513–520, 1988

Volkow ND, Fowler JS, Wolf AP, et al: Effects of chronic cocaine abuse on postsynaptic dopamine receptors. American Journal of Psychiatry 147:719–724, 1990

Wallace BC: Cocaine dependence treatment on an inpatient detoxification unit. Journal of Substance Abuse Treatment 4:85–92, 1987

Washton AM: Nonpharmacologic treatment of cocaine abuse. Psychiatric Clinics of North America 9:563–571, 1986

Weddington WW, Brown BS, Haertzen CA, et al: Changes in mood, craving, and sleep during short-term abstinence reported by male cocaine addicts. Archives of General Psychiatry 47:861–868, 1990

Weiss RD, Mirin SM: Tricyclic antidepressants in the treatment of alcoholism and drug abuse. Journal of Clinical Psychiatry 50:4–8, 1989

Weiss RD, Mirin SM: Psychological and pharmacological treatment strategies in cocaine dependence. Annals of Clinical Psychiatry 2:239–243, 1990

Weiss RD, Pope HG Jr, Mirin SM: Treatment of chronic cocaine abuse and attention deficit disorder, residual type, with magnesium pemoline. Drug and Alcohol Dependence 15:69–72, 1985

Weiss RD, Mirin SM, Michael JL, et al: Psychopathology in chronic cocaine abusers. American Journal of Drug and Alcohol Abuse 12:17–26, 1986

Weiss RD, Mirin SM, Griffin ML, et al: Psychopathology in cocaine abusers: changing trends. Journal of Nervous and Mental Disease 176:719–725, 1988

Weiss RD, Griffin ML, Mirin SM: Drug abuse as self-medication for depression: an empirical study. American Journal of Drug and Alcohol Abuse 18:121–129, 1992

Witkin G: The men who created crack. U.S. News and World Report, August 19, 1991, pp 44–53

Index

In this index, a *See* cross-reference directs you to the synonym where you can find the page numbers. A *See also* cross-reference directs you to a related topic or to a more detailed page breakdown of the topic.

Q

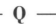

R

S